Emergencies in Psychiatry
in Low- and Middle-Income Countries

SECOND EDITION

Emergencies in Psychiatry
in Low- and Middle-Income Countries

SECOND EDITION

Edited by

R. THARA
Director
Schizophrenia Research Foundation (SCARF)
Chennai, Tamil Nadu, India

LAKSHMI VIJAYAKUMAR
Founder Trustee
SNEHA, Chennai, Tamil Nadu, India

Routledge
Taylor & Francis Group
NEW YORK AND LONDON

BYWORD BOOKS™

Second edition published 2017
by Routledge
711 Third Avenue, New York, NY 10017

and by Routledge
2 Park Square, Milton Park, Abingdon, Oxon, OX14 4RN

Routledge is an imprint of the Taylor & Francis Group, an informa business

First edition published 2012 by Byword Books Private Limited

Library of Congress Cataloging-in-Publication Data
A catalog record for this book has been requested

ISBN: 978-1-138-30019-4 (hbk)
ISBN: 978-1-4987-6714-9 (pbk)
ISBN: 978-1-315-38125-1 (ebk)

Typeset in Times, Optima
by Jacob Thomas, New Delhi, India
Cover design: Netra Shyam

Contents

Foreword

In many low-income countries, psychiatrists are so few that they unavoidably spend much of their time dealing with emergency situations. They may be called on to intervene by other physicians or clinical officers, by the police, by relatives or spouses, by teachers or other staff in school settings, by traditional healers, or in some tourist areas, even by the personnel of hotels or resorts where foreigners are lodged. In several areas of the world, emergency interventions by psychiatrists are increasingly being sought by those affected by war, disasters, and forced migration.

This book provides a comprehensive picture of the various situations in which an emergency intervention by a psychiatrist may be called for. Special attention has been paid to the context of the emergencies, the differential diagnoses of the psychiatric states, the modalities through which the interventions must be implemented, as well as the nature of these interventions. An attempt has been made to consider the legal context, with special regard to the regulations for compulsory admission, and the cultural component, especially in the case of family and school emergencies.

The emerging awareness of the multiple interrelationships between mental and physical diseases, and their relevance in the area of emergencies, is appropriately reflected in the volume, as is the frequent and powerful role of substance abuse in a variety of emergency situations.

I particularly appreciated the careful handling of the issue of violence and aggression, which is so frequently involved in appropriate as well as inappropriate calls for urgent psychiatric assessment and intervention. Especially in urban hospital settings, it seems that every patient who happens to be aggressive for any reason becomes a candidate for a psychiatric consultation. The experienced psychiatrist is well aware of this, and of the need to educate his medical colleagues on the nature and boundaries of the mandate of our profession. Probably less diffuse is the awareness of the frequent occurrence of social emergencies in the community, especially within families, that psychiatrists may be called on to deal with in settings in which community mental health is well developed, and which may need a lot of expertise and knowledge of the local cultural context.

I think this volume, which is written in simple language and provides a number of well-constructed tables and boxes, conveys many of the complexities of dealing with psychiatric emergencies. I believe it represents an extremely valuable tool for front-line clinicians in all areas of the world.

MARIO MAJ
(Former President, World Psychiatric Association)
Department of Psychiatry, University of Naples SUN, Naples, Italy

Preface to the Second Edition

Psychiatric emergencies are situations in which the patient may act in a manner that is dangerous to themselves or to others. Up to 5% of patients attending emergency departments present with primary psychiatric conditions, and a further 20%–30% have psychiatric symptoms in addition to physical disorders.

Although a majority (around 80%) of the global population lives in low- and middle-income countries, the human and fiscal resources allotted to mental healthcare in these countries are grossly inadequate. As a result of the social stigma attached to mental disorders, together with the pressure to tackle the more urgent medical healthcare needs in developing countries, psychiatric care is accorded relatively lower priority. The social costs of mental disorders, for example, to families, social welfare or criminal justice systems, are also likely to be enormous. Nevertheless, the past decade has witnessed a phenomenal growth in the evidence base on mental health in these countries.

One of the cardinal facets of the delivery of mental healthcare is the attention given to emergency conditions – which is the focus of this book. The manifestations of psychiatric emergencies in developing countries may be colored by many factors, such as culture, the social context, and religious belief systems. Hence, there is a need to not only understand these, but also formulate logical and acceptable forms of intervention. This book attempts to give the reader an overview of the kinds of psychiatric emergencies that can occur and the strategies employed to manage these in developing countries.

This book covers various areas of emergency psychiatry in the context of the developing world. The chapters on anxiety disorders, psychotic disorders, personality disorders, and substance abuse disorders describe the presentation and management of these disorders in the emergency setting. The book also deals with special population groups, such as women, children, and the elderly, who require different modes of intervention. As these groups constitute a vulnerable population in developing countries, the chapters dealing with them highlight the need for a special process of evaluation and intervention. The next group of chapters addresses emergencies following psychosocial and environmental events. Among the aspects covered are grief, suicidal behavior, and psychiatric emergencies following disasters. These chapters have a special significance, considering the rising rate of suicide and increase in the frequency of disasters in developing countries. The chapters on suicidal and uncooperative patients dwell on particularly challenging clinical situations, emphasizing ethical issues and the need to ensure the safety of the patient. A discussion of the medicolegal aspects of a psychiatric emergency in developing countries is of relevance since many countries still follow outdated and archaic legal procedures. As patients often present to the emergency department both with psychiatric as well as physical symptoms, a few chapters are devoted to psychiatric emergencies associated with medical disorders, sexual disorders, and drug-related issues.

The second edition of the book has an additional and very important chapter on emergencies associated with terrorism.

In recent decades, there has been a dramatic increase in the number of psychiatric emergencies and crises in developing countries. Those providing care during the emergency situation must aim not only to deal with the crisis, but also establish acceptance and trust in the healthcare system. This book aims to meet the needs of physicians, researchers, and all emergency care personnel dealing with those in a state of emotional crisis. It should serve to help all types of mental health professionals in developing countries to effectively and appropriately manage the various kinds of psychiatric emergencies.

We thank all the authors from around the world who so willingly agreed to contribute to this volume. We also thank Professor Mario Maj for his wonderful Foreword.

R. THARA
LAKSHMI VIJAYAKUMAR
Chennai, India

December 2016

Contributors

Olurotimi Adejumo
Centre for Child and Adolescent Mental Health (CCAMH), University of Ibadan, Ibadan, Nigeria; radejumo@yahoo.com

Atul Ambekar
National Drug Dependence Treatment Centre and Department of Psychiatry
All India Institute of Medical Sciences, New Delhi, India
atul.ambekar@gmail.com

Nargis Asad
Department of Psychiatry, Aga Khan University, Stadium Road, Karachi 74800, Pakistan; nargis.asad@aku.edu

Tolulope Bella
Centre for Child and Adolescent Mental Health (CCAMH), University of Ibadan, Ibadan, Nigeria; bellatt2002@yahoo.com

Vivek Benegal
Centre for Addiction Medicine, National Institute of Mental health and Neurosciences (NIMHANS), Bengaluru 560029, Karnataka, India
vbenegal@gmail.com

Hamid Dabholkar
Parivartan, Satara, Maharashtra, India; hamid.dabholkar@gmail.com

Julian Eaton
London School of Hygiene and Tropical Medicine, London, UK
julian.eaton@cbm.org

Nishant Goyal
Centre for Cognitive Neurosciences, Central Institute of Psychiatry, Ranchi, Jharkhand, India; psynishant@gmail.com

Sandeep Grover
Department of Psychiatry, Postgraduate Institute of Medical Education and Research (PGIMER), Chandigarh 160012, India; drsandeepg2002@yahoo.com

Patricia Ibeziako
Department of Psychiatry, Children's Hospital Boston and Harvard Medical School Boston MA, USA; Patricia.Ibeziako@childrens.harvard.edu

K.S. Jacob
Department of Psychiatry, Christian Medical College, Vellore 632002, Tamil Nadu, India; ksjacob@cmcvellore.ac.in

Shaji K.S.
Department of Psychiatry, Medical College, Thrissur 680596, Kerala, India drshajiks@gmail.com

Gurvinder Kalra
Staff Psychiatrist, Latrobe Regional Hospital (LRH), LRH Mental Health Services, Victoria 3844, Australia; kalragurvinder@gmail.com

Murad Moosa Khan
Department of Psychiatry, Aga Khan University, Stadium Road, Karachi 74800, Pakistan; murad.khan@aku.edu

Parmanand Kulhara
Department of Psychiatry, Postgraduate Institute of Medical Education and Research (PGIMER), Chandigarh 160012, India; param_kulhara@yahoo.co.in

T.C. Ramesh Kumar
Schizophrenia Research Foundation (SCARF), Anna Nagar, Chennai 600101, Tamil Nadu, India; rameshkumar@scarfindia.org

Anju Kuruvilla
Department of Psychiatry, Christian Medical College, Vellore 632002, Tamil Nadu, India; sanju@cmcvellore.ac.in

Ilyas Mirza
Barnet Enfield and Haringey Mental Health NHS Trust, UK and Principal Research Scientist, Human Development Research Foundation, Pakistan; iqmirza@gmail.com

Tania Nadeem
Department of Psychiatry, Aga Khan University, Stadium Road, Karachi 74800, Pakistan; tania.nadeem@aku.edu

Juliet E.M. Nakku
Department of Psychiatry, Makerere University College of Health Sciences, Butabika National Referral and Teaching Hospital, P.O. Box 7017, Kampala, Uganda; jnakku@yahoo.com

Janardhanan C. Narayanaswamy
Department of Psychiatry, National Institute of Mental health and Neurosciences (NIMHANS), Bengaluru 560029, Karnataka, India; jairamnimhans@gmail.com

S. Haque Nizamie
Central Institute of Psychiatry, Kanke (PO), Ranchi 834006, Jharkhand, India
sh.nizamie@gmail.com

Olayinka Omigbodun
Centre for Child and Adolescent Mental Health (CCAMH), University of Ibadan, Ibadan, Nigeria; olayinka.omigbodun@gmail.com

R. Padmavati
Schizophrenia Research Foundation (SCARF), Anna Nagar, Chennai 600101, Tamil Nadu, India; padmavati@scarfindia.org

Atif Rahman
Institute of Psychology, Health and Society, University of Liverpool, UK
Atif.rahman@liverpool.ac.uk

T.S. Sathyanarayana Rao
Department of Psychiatry, JSS Medical College, Mysore 570004, Karnataka, India
tssrao19@gmail.com, tssrao19@yahoo.com

Anoop Raveendran
Department of Psychiatry, Christian Medical College, Vellore 632002, Tamil Nadu, India; anoopsych@gmail.com

Y.C. Janardhan Reddy
Department of Psychiatry, National Institute of Mental health and Neurosciences (NIMHANS), Bengaluru 560029, Karnataka, India; ycjreddy@gmail.com

Athula Sumathipala
Institute of Psychiatry, King's College London, Box P036, De Crespigny Park, London SE5 8AF, United Kingdom; athula.sumathipala@kcl.ac.uk

Sumesh T.P.
Department of Psychiatry, Medical College, Thrissur 680596, Kerala, India

Hema Tharoor
Schizophrenia Research Foundation (SCARF), Anna Nagar, Chennai 600101, Tamil Nadu, India; hematharoor@scarfindia.org

Sai Krishna Tikka
Central Institute of Psychiatry, Ranchi, Jharkhand, India; cricsai@gmail.com

Lakshmi Vijayakumar
Founder Trustee, Sneha, Chennai, Tamil Nadu, India; lakshmi@vijayakumars.com

Vinayak Vijayakumar
Sneha, Chennai, Tamil Nadu, India; vinayak@vijayakumars.com

Lopa Winters
Whittington Hospital, London, UK; lopa.winters@nhs.net

Abbreviations

ACE	angiotensin-converting enzyme
ADHD	attention deficit hyperactivity disorder
AIDS	acquired immune deficiency syndrome
APA	American Psychiatric Association
ARDSI	Alzheimer's and Related Disorders Society of India
ATSM	acute traumatic stress management
BPSD	behavioral and psychological symptoms of dementia
CAMH	child and adolescent mental health
CBT	cognitive behavioral therapy
CDC	Centers for Disease Control and Prevention
CISM	critical incident stress management
CSF	cerebrospinal fluid
CVA	cerebral vascular accident
DT	delirium tremens
ECG	electrocardiogram
ECT	electroconvulsive therapy
ED	emergency department
EEG	electroencephalogram
ER	emergency room
GABA	gamma-aminobutyric acid
GAD	generalized anxiety disorder
GHB	gamma-hydroxy butyrate
HAART	highly active antiretroviral therapy
ICD	International Classification of Disease
ICIVAD	intracavernosal injection of vasoactive drugs
LAAM	levo-alpha acetyl methadol
LAMI	low- and middle-income (countries)
mhGAP	Mental Health Gap Action Programme
MR/DD	mental retardation and development disabilities
NICE	National Institute for Health and Care Excellence
NNRTI	non-nucleoside reverse transcriptase inhibitor
NSAID	non-steroidal anti-inflammatory drug
OCD	obsessive–compulsive disorder
OPD	outpatient department
PCB	polychlorinated biphenyl
PDE	phosphodiesterase
PFA	psychological first aid

PIPE	Psychiatrists In-Practice Examination
PTG	post-traumatic growth
PTSD	post-traumatic stress disorder
RT	rapid tranquilization
SIADH	syndrome of inappropriate antidiuretic hormone secretion
SIB	self-injurious behavior
SNRI	serotonin and norepinephrine reuptake inhibitor
SSRI	selective serotonin reuptake inhibitor
TB	tuberculosis
TCA	tricyclic antidepressant
TIA	transient ischemic attack
VFB	vaginal foreign bodies
WHO	World Health Organization

1 Anxious Patient in the Emergency Ward

Janardhanan C. Narayanaswamy,
Y.C. Janardhan Reddy

INTRODUCTION

Anxiety, a common problem encountered in psychiatric emergency services, is defined as an unpleasant emotional state consisting of psychophysiological responses to the anticipation of real or imagined danger. Fear can be distinguished from anxiety in that it is a clear response to a threat that is definitely from an external source. Anxiety is possibly an adaptation mechanism or a survival cue, according to the evolutionary hypothesis. It can be considered a normal and adaptive response that has life-saving qualities. It prompts a person to take necessary steps to prevent the threat or lessen its consequences. When a person is faced with a stressful situation, a heightened autonomic discharge occurs. When this becomes intense, inappropriate, or miscued, anxiety symptoms result. Even though anxiety may not be directly associated with life-threatening consequences, the burden it carries in the form of social and occupational dysfunction is enormous, and hence it mandates prompt management in emergency settings. There is a need for the emergency clinician or psychiatrist to liaison with physicians and cardiologists for optimal clinical care. After the initial management of the crisis in the emergency services, the clinician is urged to make necessary arrangements for continuing care in the long term.

PRESENTATION IN EMERGENCY SERVICES

A patient suffering from anxiety could present to the emergency clinician with a wide variety of symptoms, ranging from somatic symptoms to severe agitation. Anxiety has physiological, physical, and cognitive manifestations. The cognitive or psychological component is related to the thinking of the person at the time when he or she is suffering from anxiety. The person could, for example, be fearing scrutiny by others, fearing impending doom, etc. The physical component of anxiety consists of muscle tension or fidgetiness, while the physiological symptoms are autonomic symptoms, such as palpitation, sweating, and diarrhea. It is important to check for all dimensions of the symptoms since the patient could present with a predominant dimension, such as physical or physiological symptoms. Figure 1.1 shows the major symptoms of anxiety.

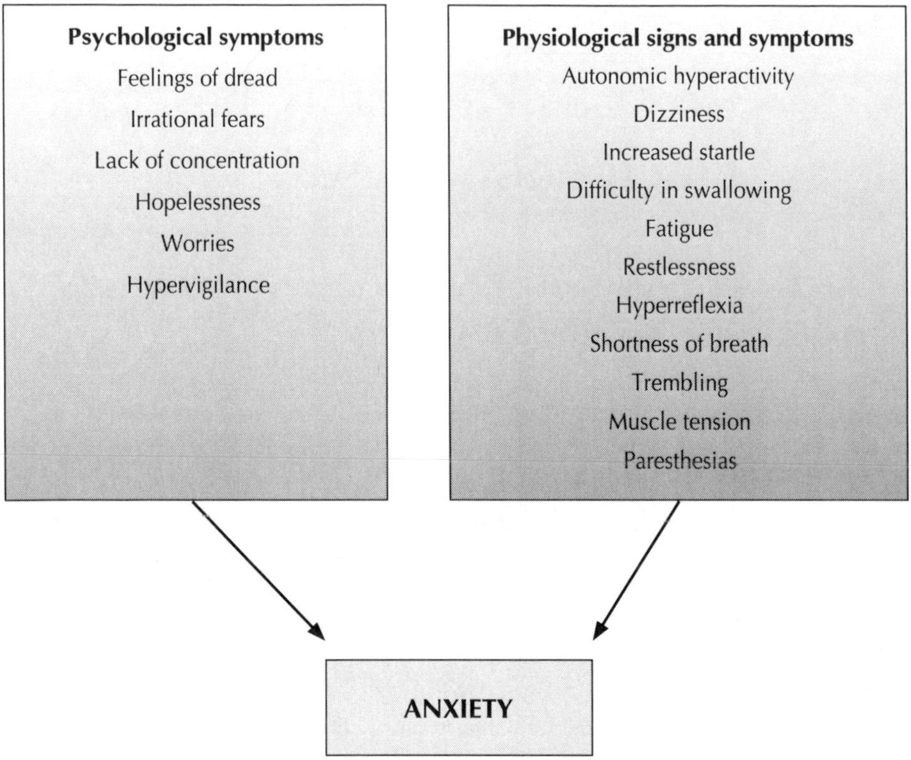

Figure 1.1 The constellation of anxiety symptoms

A significant proportion of patients with anxiety symptoms seek treatment in general hospital settings. Hence, it is imperative that there is a good liaison system in place. It demands a continuous dialogue between the emergency clinician and the psychiatrist, cardiologist, respiratory medicine specialist, physician, etc. This is crucial since there is a need to rule out serious medical concerns that might simulate or be associated with anxiety. Conversely, many medical disorders such as bronchial asthma and cardiac conditions might be associated with prominent anxiety symptoms, making it essential to liaison with a psychiatrist.

Irrespective of the underlying causes of their anxiety, the majority of patients present with the physiological and sometimes the physical symptoms, as these are perceived to be distressing and alarming. These symptoms can be misleading and may result in many patients seeking treatment in a medical emergency unit. For example, anxious patients with prominent palpitations and sweating might seek treatment in a cardiac/medical emergency unit, fearing that they have a catastrophic cardiac illness. Nonetheless, one needs to keep in mind that the manifestations of anxiety are often accompanied by medical illnesses (Petit 2004; Khouzam, Tan and Gill 2008). The emergency ward clinician or psychiatrist must be aware of the medical conditions that may accompany the manifestations of anxiety, and must attentively consider such possibilities by meticulously noting down the patient's history, so that prompt action can be taken. Table 1.1 lists the medical conditions that may accompany the prominent

TABLE 1.1

Medical Conditions Associated with Anxiety Symptoms

- *Endocrine causes*
  Hyperthyroidism, pheochromocytoma, parathyroid dysfunction, premenstrual syndrome, carcinoids
- *Cardiac causes*
  Myocardial infarction and anginas, arrhythmias, hypovolemia, hypertension, congestive heart failure, syncope, hypertension, valvular diseases
- *Respiratory conditions*
  Acute bronchial asthma, chronic obstructive pulmonary disease, pulmonary embolism, pulmonary edema, pneumothorax, sleep apnea
- *Neurological conditions*
  Cerebrovascular accidents, seizures, migraine, vestibular dysfunctions, myasthenia
- *Metabolic conditions*
  Hypoglycemia, hyponatremia, hyperkalemia, porphyrias
- *Drug- and substance-related*
  Substance intoxication and withdrawal (such as alcohol, opioids, stimulants, hypnotic sedatives), akathisia due to dopaminergics, anticholinergics-related, sympathomimetics, bronchodilators

symptoms of anxiety.

An anxiety syndrome of new and acute onset merits a detailed evaluation of the medical and psychiatric causes. Once the medical conditions have been excluded, the patient's psychiatric history should be elicited meticulously for delineation of the anxiety syndrome. In such a case, the common diagnoses to be considered are:

- Generalized anxiety disorder
- Panic disorder
- Social anxiety/phobia
- Acute stress disorder
- Post-traumatic stress disorder (PTSD)
- Obsessive–compulsive disorder

Generalized Anxiety Disorder

A patient suffering from generalized anxiety disorder (GAD) must have the primary symptoms of anxiety on most days for at least several weeks at a time, and usually for several months (at least 6 months) (American Psychiatric Association 2013). The principal symptoms of GAD are "excessive anxiety and worry" about a variety of events and situations, difficulty in controlling anxiety and worry, along with restlessness or feeling keyed up or on edge. In addition, the person is easily fatigued, has difficulty concentrating or mind goes blank, and there is irritability, muscle tension, and sleep disturbances.

Patients with GAD often have physical symptoms and it may be difficult to distinguish these from those of medical illnesses that are associated with anxiety. Factors suggesting that the anxiety is the symptom of a medical disorder include the onset of the symptoms at a later age, no personal or family history of anxiety, no increase in stress, little or no avoidance of anxiety-provoking situations, and a poor response to anti-anxiety medication. A physical cause should be suspected when the anxiety follows recent changes in medication or accompanies signs and symptoms of a new disease (Katon 2006).

The anxiety, worry, or physical symptoms cause clinically significant distress or impairment in social, occupational or other important areas of functioning. More than two-thirds of GAD patients have one or more comorbid psychiatric disorders, of which social phobia, depression, and panic disorder are the most common.

Panic Disorder

Panic disorder is characterized by the recurrent occurrence of panic attacks that are marked by severe anxiety and which are not restricted to any particular situation or set of circumstances and are, therefore, unpredictable (Katon 2006). Individual attacks last only a few minutes, though the duration and frequency vary. The person experiences a crescendo of fear and autonomic symptoms which drive them to leave wherever they may be. Patients of panic disorder typically report experiencing a sense of impending doom and feelings such as "I am going to die" and "I will go crazy" at the time of the attacks. Anticipatory anxiety is a prominent feature and patients worry about the consequences of recurrent attacks. Panic attacks are not unique to panic disorder and can occur in other anxiety disorders as well. They could even be due to medical conditions or substances. In cases where the panic attack occurs in an established phobic situation, phobia should be given diagnostic preference. Panic attacks may be secondary to depression, and if the criteria for depression are fulfilled at the same time, then panic disorder should not be given as the main diagnosis.

The frightening physical symptoms of panic disorder often lead to the extensive use of medical services. Patients with medically unexplained syndromes, such as irritable bowel syndrome, chest pain with negative results on cardiac testing, palpitations, interstitial cystitis, and chronic fatigue syndrome, have been shown to have higher rates of coexisting panic disorder than do control subjects with documented medical syndromes. The frequency of panic disorder is also higher among patients with bronchial asthma, mitral-valve prolapse, labile hypertension, and migraine than among those without these conditions (Katon 2006). It is essential to take the patient's history carefully and conduct a physical examination to rule out medical causes of the symptoms. Conditions and agents that can mimic or cause panic attacks include thyroid abnormalities, neurological conditions such as temporal-lobe epilepsy, bronchial asthma, cardiac arrhythmias, pheochromocytoma, excessive intake of stimulants including caffeine, withdrawal from psychoactive substances and alcohol, and treatment with corticosteroids. Biochemical investigations, measurement of thyrotropin levels, and electrocardiography are often ordered to identify any underlying medical causes, but these tests usually have negative results in the absence of other evidence suggesting medical causes. Screening for depression is also important because of its increased prevalence among patients with panic disorder and the associated risk of suicidal behavior (Pollack and Marzol 2000).

Social Phobia/Anxiety

Social anxiety disorder, also known as social phobia, is one of the most common psychiatric disorders. Its onset is usually during childhood or adolescence. The typical feature of social phobia is a marked and persistent fear of one or more social or performance-related situations, in which the person is exposed to unfamiliar people or to possible scrutiny by others (American Psychiatric Association 2013). The individual fears that he or she will act in a way (or show anxiety symptoms) that will be humiliating or embarrassing. The person recognizes that the fear is excessive or unreasonable. Exposure to the feared social situation almost invariably provokes anxiety, which may take the form of a panic attack. The person avoids the feared social or performance-related situations or endures them with intense anxiety or distress. Social phobia is of two subtypes – generalized and non-generalized/circumscribed. In the generalized type, the person experiences anxiety during most social situations or avoids these situations. In the circumscribed type, anxiety occurs only in specific social situations (e.g. public speaking) (American Psychiatric Association 2013; Schneier 2006). Social anxiety disorder differs from shyness and performance anxiety in that its severity, pervasiveness, and the resultant distress and impairment are greater. Persons with social anxiety disorder may avoid important activities, such as attending classes and meetings, or attend them but avoid active participation. Anticipatory anxiety is common.

Screening questions regarding avoidance of embarrassment, avoidance of being the centre of attention, and fear of being embarrassed or looking stupid have high sensitivity and specificity for the generalized type of social anxiety disorder, and positive responses indicating fear and avoidance should be followed by further inquiry. Many fear that others will notice their physical manifestations of anxiety, such as sweating, trembling and blushing, and they overestimate the visibility of these features. Panic attacks may occur in social anxiety disorder, but unlike those in panic disorder, these attacks occur only in relation to current or anticipated social situations. Though worry and symptoms of anxiety are characteristic of GAD as well, in social anxiety disorder these features are associated predominantly with social situations. There can be high comorbidity with depression, other anxiety disorders, and substance use.

Acute Stress Disorder and Post-traumatic Stress Disorder

Acute stress disorder can develop within one month of exposure to a traumatic event, the prominent symptoms being anxiety and increased arousal. The person's response involves intense fear and a sense of horror and helplessness. The traumatic event is persistently experienced in recurrent thoughts, images, and dreams. The symptoms mentioned above should last for at least two days and a maximum of four weeks, and should develop within one month of the occurrence of the traumatic event (American Psychiatric Association 2013). If the symptoms develop after one month, the possibility of post-traumatic stress disorder needs to be considered.

Obsessive–Compulsive Disorder (OCD)

The clinical picture of OCD is characterized by obsessions and compulsions (American Psychiatric Association 2013; World Health Organization 1992). Even though strictly OCD is not discussed under the rubric of anxiety disorders, the condition is characterized by prominent anxiety symptoms. Obsessions are recurrent, intrusive, unwanted, and persistent thoughts/urges. These are recognized as originating from the person's own mind, but cause significant anxiety or distress. The person tries to offer resistance to these thoughts, but feels that they are too overpowering and difficult to control. In response to obsessions, the person gives in to compulsions, which are repetitive motor or mental acts aimed at reducing anxiety or preventing certain undesired outcomes. Patients with OCD usually have good insight (even though a subgroup has been shown to have poor insight), and realize that their behavior is illogical and senseless. The obsessions center around many themes (Leckman *et al.* 1997) but there are some common ones. The common obsessions are fear of contamination or contracting an illness, doubts about daily activities, unwanted thoughts related to sex, harm, and religion, and a need for symmetry. The common compulsions are washing and cleaning, checking, repetition, arranging things, and mental rituals or compulsions (e.g. praying, counting, and contrast thinking).

The likelihood of diagnosis is greatly increased by routine screening questions such as: "Do you have repetitive thoughts which cause anxiety but which you are not able to ward off regardless of how hard you try?", "Do you keep things extremely clean or wash your hands frequently?", and "Do you check things excessively?" An affirmative answer to any of these questions suggests a diagnosis of OCD, which would necessitate asking further questions on other obsessions with other themes (Jenike 2004).

ASSESSMENT OF A PATIENT WITH ANXIETY

Any new-onset anxiety symptoms merit detailed assessment.

- Anxiety can be a symptom of medical or neurological illnesses or a manifestation of substance abuse or withdrawal. Therefore, a detailed medical/neurological workup is essential. It may be necessary to take a full history and conduct screening for drugs.
- While it is important to rule out an organic basis of anxiety, unwarranted investigations may increase the patient's anxiety further; therefore, investigations have to be ordered judiciously.
- It is important to determine the cause of the anxiety once medical causes have been ruled out. Anxiety can be a symptom of anxiety disorder, depression, or even psychosis.

PHYSICAL EXAMINATION

A general physical examination should be carried out meticulously. The examination may help calm the patient down and be of use in uncovering illnesses such as a thyroid abnormality. Tremors are a very common symptom among those going through substance withdrawal. Initially, one needs to examine the vital signs such as the pulse rate, blood pressure, and respiratory rate. The presence of tachycardia, tachypnea, sweating, and other autonomic signs is common to anxiety and medical conditions. A raised resting pulse may point to hyperthyroidism, as may diastolic hypertension and eye signs. Endocrine disorders such as hyperthyroidism and hypothyroidism, pheochromocytoma, hyperadrenocorticism, and hyperparathyroidism may mimic anxiety disorders, but may also have clinching clinical features which may be obtained from the history and physical examination. Hypoglycemia is a very common condition mimicking anxiety symptoms similar to those seen in panic attacks.

Cardiovascular disorders are among the common but serious differential diagnoses. Anemia may be associated with palpitations but other features may be absent. Acute chest pain and acute myocardial infarction are associated with many symptoms of anxiety, and hence an ECG may be required to rule out these conditions. Other factors associated with these conditions also help in confirming or ruling them out. Supraventricular arrhythmias are usually associated with a funny sensation in the chest and may mimic anxiety disorders, but the ECG is diagnostic. Chronic lung disorders may be associated with secondary arrthymias and may mimic anxiety disorder. Among the neurological causes, seizures (especially complex partial seizure) may have anxiety symptoms as a part of the prodrome or aura. Similarly, severe movement disorders such as Parkinson disease and acute-onset vascular events such as transient ischemic attack (TIA), and cerebrovascular accident (CVA) are accompanied by anxiety symptoms.

The side-effects of drugs or medications ought to be an important consideration in a psychiatry emergency. Akathisia caused by the use of antipsychotics may be a relatively common condition among those presenting to the emergency ward (Petit 2004). The intense restlessness and subjective inner discomfort may simulate anxiety symptoms. Acute dystonic reactions are also associated with overwhelming anxiety due to the alarming nature of the condition. The findings of an examination would clinch the diagnosis quite easily. Similarly, selective serotonin reuptake inhibitor (SSRI)-induced anxiety (activation symptoms) (Zinner 1994; Bernstein 2006) is common in the first few weeks of starting these drugs. Caffeine, monosodium glutamate (Chinese restaurant syndrome), and a variety of drugs that are abused can cause features of anxiety during intoxication or withdrawal.

MENTAL STATUS EXAMINATION

The patient's appearance, facial expression, postures, and gestures are usually suggestive of anxiety. Additional features are sweating, tremulousness, agitation, and restlessness. The thought processes are usually normal, even though there are worries and the patient anticipates a catastrophic outcome. The mood is usually marked by anxiety. There could be perceptual disturbances if the patient uses psychoactive substances or has a psychotic disorder. Derealization and depersonalization could be present as markers of intense anxiety. Anxiety can also be a feature of delirium in which a predominant feature is altered sensorium. Severe forms of anxiety are associated with prominent psychomotor changes, which could make the patient agitated. Insight and judgment depend on the level of distress.

MANAGEMENT

Medical causes need to be treated in patients with medical conditions. It is of the utmost importance to have a good liaison with the medical emergency unit (Petit 2004). The clinician should be alert and consider various medical possibilities rather than arriving at a psychiatric diagnosis directly. The treatment should focus on the suspected psychiatric disorder rather than the symptoms. The clinician should put the patients at ease by talking to them and reassuring them in order to allay their anxiety. This is important because the very fact of being in an emergency setting might provoke anxiety. The clinician must take a detailed history, and acute emergency care must be instituted with the aim of reducing acute symptoms.

Benzodiazepines

In the emergency setting, benzodiazepines are the best short-acting drugs (Bernstein *et al.* 2006). Benzodiazepines are a large class of relatively safe and widely prescribed medications that have rapid and profound anti-anxiety and sedative-hypnotic effects (Table 1.2). They are thought to exert their therapeutic effects by enhancing the inhibitory neurotransmitter systems, utilizing gamma-aminobutyric acid (GABA). The benzodiazepines most widely prescribed for the treatment of anxiety disorders are diazepam, lorazepam, clonazepam, and alprazolam. Among these agents, alprazolam and lorazepam have shorter elimination half-lives, whereas diazepam and clonazepam have a longer period of action. With continued use, benzodiazepines have the potential for producing physiological dependence. A short course of benzodiazepines may be effective in the short term and may not cause many side-effects. For instance, lorazepam at a dosage of 0.5–2 mg, given orally or intramuscularly, may provide rapid relief (Khouzam, Tan and Gill 2008). Lorazepam is often the drug of choice

TABLE 1.2

Commonly Used Benzodiazepines

Name	Initial dose (mg)	Dosage (mg)	Onset after oral dose	Dose equivalents (mg)	Elimination half-life (hour)*
Alprazolam	0.25–0.5	1–6	Intermediate	0.5	6–20
Lorazepam	0.5–1	1–10	Intermediate	1.0	10–20
Clonazepam	0.25–0.5	0.5–4	Intermediate	0.25	18–50
Oxazepam	15	30–120	Intermediate to slow	15	8–12
Diazepam	5–10	5–40	Rapid	5	30–100
Chlordiazepoxide	5–10	5–00	Intermediate	10	30–100
Temazepam	15	30–120	Intermediate	30	8–20

* Total for all active metabolites

for acute anxiety since it is well absorbed and has a rapid onset of action. Although benzodiazepines are the preferred option for acute anxiety and are relatively safe, the following important points have to be kept in mind.

- Short courses of benzodiazepines are relatively safe and such courses (up to 2–4 weeks) probably do not have addictive potential (Khouzam, Tan and Gill 2008), but long-term use may cause difficulty in withdrawal and lead to dependence. Therefore, benzodiazepines should soon be replaced by antidepressants.
- Caution should be exercised in the case of the elderly population and patients with medical/neurological disorders as benzodiazepines put them at risk of side-effects such as respiratory depression.
- Benzodiazepines may be associated with impairment of the memory, disorientation, confusion, and psychomotor disturbances.
- The use of benzodiazepines might lead to behavior disinhibition.
- Hepatic dysfunction and concomitant prescription of certain other medications can affect the metabolism of certain benzodiazepines. Lorazepam and oxazepam are less affected by these interactions.
- The use of benzodiazepines in the first trimester of pregnancy may be associated with fetal malformations, such as alimentary tract defects.

Antidepressants

Selective serotonin reuptake inhibitors (SSRIs) are currently the treatment of choice for anxiety disorders due to their efficacy and favorable side-effect profile, even though the anti-anxiety property of tricyclic antidepressants is equally effective. SSRIs should be started at a low dosage, which should be increased slowly, or they may themselves worsen the anxiety. Worsening of anxiety symptoms with SSRIs is typically seen in panic disorder. SSRIs can be initiated once the acute symptoms are better or along with benzodiazepines (Khouzam, Tan and Gill 2008). The majority of anxiety disorders respond to conventional antidepressant dosages of SSRIs. However, for OCD, a higher dosage of SSRIs is recommended. Table 1.3 lists some of the antidepressants commonly used for the treatment of anxiety disorders. Antidepressants take at least 4 weeks to become effective, though clinically, improvement is sometimes noticed within 2 weeks. They are started at a low dosage, which is increased gradually (Bernstein *et al.* 2006). It is good practice to initially give a combination of a benzodiazepine such as clonazepam (0.5–1 mg per day) and an SSRI. It is recommended that the benzodiazepine be gradually withdrawn after 1–2 months of stability in the clinical status and the patient be maintained only on an SSRI.

Another group of antidepressants called serotonin and norepinephrine reuptake inhibitors (SNRIs) is also useful in the treatment of anxiety disorders. The medications under this category are venlafaxine (75–150 mg) and duloxetine (20–40 mg). Recently, pregabalin, a novel psychotropic drug with anticonvulsant, anxiolytic, and analgesic properties, has been evaluated and has been found to be useful in GAD. Its mechanism of action is largely unknown, although it binds to an auxiliary subunit ($\alpha 2\delta$ of voltage-gated calcium channels), thereby increasing whole brain GABA. It is given at a dosage

TABLE 1.3

Antidepressants in Anxiety Disorders

Medication	Initial dose (mg)	Target dose (mg)
Selective serotonin reuptake inhibitors (SSRIs)		
Sertraline	50	100–150
Paroxetine	10	30–50
Escitalopram	05	10–20
Fluvoxamine	50	100–200
Fluoxetine	20	20–40
Tricyclics		
Amitriptyline	25	150–200
Imipramine	25	150–200
Serotonin and norepinephrine reuptake inhibitors (SNRIs)		
Venlafaxine	75	150–225
Duloxetine	20	40–60
Monoamine oxidase inhibitors		
Phenelzine	15	30–60
Other antidepressants		
Mirtazapine	15	30–45

of between 150 mg and 300 mg per day.

Buspirone, a non-benzodiazepine anxiolytic that has partial agonist properties at 5-HT1A receptors, does not have the side-effects associated with the benzodiazepines, such as sedation, impairment of memory, slowed reaction time, or physiological dependence (Bernstein *et al.* 2006). Its anti-anxiety action is of delayed onset (a few weeks). It has a short half-life and thus requires multiple daily dosing (10–30 mg per day in 2–3 divided doses).

A plan regarding the long-term care of the patient needs to be formulated in the emergency department itself. The emergency team can discuss the long-term treatment plan with the patient once relief from the symptoms has been obtained. Referral to a psychiatrist or psychologist in the outpatient department may be necessary for further follow-up care. Psychological treatments, especially cognitive behavior therapy, are now a standard and effective treatment option for the long-term management of anxiety disorders. Table 1.4 presents the commonly used psychological treatments for anxiety disorders.

CONCLUSION

Anxiety disorders are not unusual in emergency medical and psychiatry settings. It is important to recognize them and treat them appropriately. Since symptoms of anxiety are also a manifestation of many medical conditions, the clinician in the emergency services should rule out possible organic causes before initiating psychiatric

TABLE 1.4

Commonly Used Psychological Treatments for Anxiety Disorder

Psychoeducation This is aimed at clarifying misconceptions and misunderstandings, and providing a biopsychosocial model. It also facilitates compliance with treatment.
Self-monitoring This is helpful both as an assessment procedure and treatment strategy. Each time the patient feels anxious, they should record when and where the anxiety began, as well as the intensity of the experience and the symptoms that were present.
Cognitive restructuring This involves observing one's automatic thoughts and becoming aware of them. This is achieved by self-monitoring, Socratic questioning, role-playing, imagery, and filling a thought record. During therapy, one has to identify the cognitive distortions, such as catastrophizing and all-or-none (black and white) thinking, and challenge the distortions.
Relaxation This helps to reduce the physiological correlates of anxiety. It also helps in broadening the focus so that the patient can consider alternatives in anxiety-provoking situations.

intervention. However, unnecessary investigations to rule out organicity may worsen the patient's anxiety further; therefore, investigations have to be ordered judiciously. It is important to reassure the patients and calm them down. An attentive hearing may go a long way in alleviating the patient's suffering. Benzodiazepines are the first-line drugs in the treatment of anxiety in the emergency setting. However, these have to be used judiciously and should be replaced with antidepressants and cognitive behavior therapy, which should be used in the long-term management of the patient.

REFERENCES

American Psychiatric Association 2013, *Diagnostic and Statistical Manual of Mental Disorders* (5th ed.). Arlington, VA: American Psychiatric Publishing.

Bernstein, CA, Levin, Z, Poag, M and Rubinstein, M 2006, *On call psychiatry*. Philadelphia: Elsevier.

Jenike, MA 2004, Clinical practice. Obsessive–compulsive disorder. *N Engl J Med,* 350, 259–265.

Katon, WJ 2006, Panic disorder. *N Engl J Med,* 354, 2360–2367.

Khouzam, HR, Tan, DT and Gill, TS 2008, *Handbook on emergency psychiatry*. Philadelphia: Mosby Elsevier.

Leckman, JF, Grice, DE, Boardman, J, Zhang, H, Vitale, A, Bondi, C, Alsobrook, J, Peterson, BS, Cohen, DJ, Rasmussen, SA, Goodman, WK, McDougle, CJ and Pauls, DL 1997, Symptoms of obsessive-compulsive disorder. *Am J Psychiatry,* 154, 911–917.

Petit, JR 2004, *Handbook of Eemergency Psychiatry*. Philadelphia: Lippincott Williams and Wilkins.

Pollack, MH and Marzol, PC 2000, Panic: Course, complications and treatment of panic disorder. *J Psychopharmacol,* 14, S25–30.

Saran, A and Halaris, A 1989, Panic attack precipitated by fluoxetine. *J Neuropsychiatry Clin Neurosci,* 1, 219–220.

Schneier, FR 2006, Clinical practice. Social anxiety disorder. *N Engl J Med,* 355, 1029–1036.

World Health Organization (WHO) 1992, The ICD classification of mental and behavioral disorders 11: Clinical description and diagnostic guidelines. Geneva: WHO.

Zinner, SH 1994, Panic attacks precipitated by sertraline. *Am J Psychiatry,* 151, 147–148.

2 Psychiatric Emergencies in Substance Abuse

Hamid Dabholkar, Atul Ambekar, Vivek Benegal

INTRODUCTION

Substance use disorders remain a low-priority area worldwide in spite of the relatively high prevalence (up to 5% in the general population) and the disproportionately huge social burden (4% of disability-adjusted life-years) caused by them (Gururaj *et al.* 2011; Benegal, Chand and Obot 2009). The scenario is more challenging in the low- and middle-income (LAMI) countries where there is continuing increase in the availability of substances (especially alcohol) and huge gaps in access to treatment (up to 80%) (Benegal, Chand and Obot 2009). Emergency services are an important component of any substance abuse treatment service. Two important settings where patients might seek help are the emergency departments (EDs) of general hospitals and those of specialty psychiatric hospitals. In addition to these settings, police and other law enforcement officers also commonly face emergencies related to substance use. Emergencies due to substance use contribute up to 3% of all emergencies in the

BOX 2.1 IMPORTANT QUESTIONS FOR EVALUATION OF A PATIENT

- What are the patient's vital signs and level of consciousness?
- Are the patient's current status and behavior an immediate threat to themselves or others?
- What are the substances that the patient may have consumed? How much and for how long? When did they last consume the substance/s?
- How are these substances affecting and likely to affect the patient's medical status and behavior at present and in the near future?
- Is the patient's condition likely to be partly or wholly due to other conditions, such as injuries or systemic illness (e.g. head injury or diabetic ketoacidosis mimicking or complicating drug intoxication)?
- Are there any medical comorbidities for which the patient is taking treatment?
- Are there any specific medicolegal aspects involved in this case?

emergency units of general hospitals (Bhalla, Datta and Chakrabarti 2006). In specialist psychiatry emergency settings, emergencies due to substance abuse contribute up to 12% of the case load (Sahoo *et al.* 2010). The substances abused by those presenting to emergency settings in LAMI countries usually include alcohol, various forms and preparations of opioids, inhalant, and volatile substances, different stimulants, sedatives–hypnotics, and benzodiazepines–anxiolytics. Multisubstance abuse is also not uncommon. Intoxication and withdrawal are the most prevalent conditions with which patients present to emergency settings. Substance-induced psychosis and anxiety disorders are other important presentations. Most of the time, patients are brought to the ED by family members and friends, but a significant number are also brought by the police and law enforcement personnel. Patients presenting with substance-related emergency is one of the most challenging situations faced by the on-call physician or psychiatrist. They not only present a management challenge because of their behavioral manifestations, but also can lead to potentially life-threatening situations (Box 2.1).

COMMON PRESENTATIONS IN EMERGENCIES RELATED TO SUBSTANCE ABUSE

Intoxication

The common substances consumed by patients presenting with intoxication and overdose to psychiatric emergency services are alcohol, opioids, anxiolytics–benzodiazepines, sedatives–hypnotics, stimulant drugs (methamphetamine, cocaine), and cannabis (Bienenfeld and Sellers 2001). Table 2.1 summarizes the signs and symptoms, together with the management protocol to be followed.

GENERAL LINES FOR MANAGEMENT OF EMERGENCIES DUE TO SUBSTANCE ABUSE (BOXES 2.2–2.3)

- Evaluate the patient in a peaceful and quiet area.
- Monitor the patient's vital signs and level of consciousness.
- Ensure hydration. Encourage the oral intake of fluids. If this is not possible, consider administering fluids intravenously.
- Adopt a supportive approach while dealing with the anxious and perplexed patient. Reassurance and explanations may be helpful.

BOX 2.2 INDICATIONS FOR INPATIENT MANAGEMENT

- Fever
- Seizures
- Protracted nausea/vomiting/diarrhea
- Altered sensorium
- Aggression or violence
- Delusions or hallucinations, with impaired reality testing
- Signs of the Wernicke–Korsakoff syndrome

TABLE 2.1

Signs and Symptoms and the Management Protocol for Emergencies Related to Substance Abuse

Name of the substance	Signs and symptoms	Management
Alcohol	Smell of alcohol, disinhibition, slurred speech, agitation, restlessness, ataxia, conjunctival congestion, tachycardia, hypertension, nystagmus, coma	Caution should be observed with respect to potential aggression and violence. Any such aggression can be treated with intramuscular haloperidol (5–10 mg) and/or lorazepam (1–2 mg). Fifty milliliters of 50% glucose may be administered if hypoglycemia is suspected. Patients with a history of alcohol dependence syndrome should be given thiamine (100 mg) intramuscularly and then orally for 6 days to prevent the onset of Wernicke encephalopathy.
Methanol poisoning	Initially, complaints of nausea, dizziness, headache, lack of coordination, and confusion. Sufficiently large doses cause unconsciousness and death. Initial symptoms wane and people are lulled into thinking that they have improved. But a second set of symptoms arises, 10–30 hours after the initial exposure, which include blurring or complete loss of vision, and acidosis, leading to death by respiratory failure	Acidosis to be corrected with intravenous sodium bicarbonate, the further generation of toxic metabolite should be blocked till patient can be transported to hospital for dialysis, by administration of (i) fomepizole – loading dose of 15 mg/kg, followed by 10 mg/kg every 12 hours for 4 doses, followed by 15 mg/kg every 12 hours till serum methanol concentration is <20 mg/dL; or (ii) ethanol – oral solution of 42.8% v/v spirits – loading dose of 2 mL/kg, followed by 0.5 mL/kg/hour.
Opioids	Pinpoint pupils unresponsive to light, depressed respiration and level of consciousness, bradycardia, hypothermia, pulmonary edema	Treat with intravenous naloxone (0.4–2.0 mg) every 2–3 minutes until respiration is stable. After 10 mg, consider other causes for symptomatology. The half-life of naloxone is much shorter than that of most opioids (approximately 1 hour), so observe the patient closely for the re-emergence of symptoms (e.g. coma) and retreat with naloxone. The failure to do so may result in the patient's death after release from the emergency room.

(continued)

TABLE 2.1 (*continued*)

Name of the substance	Signs and symptoms	Management
Sedatives–hypnotics	Ataxia, slurred speech, nystagmus, confusion, decreased respiration, decreased level of consciousness, hypotension	Perform gastric lavage if the drug was taken in the last 4–6 hours. Forced diuresis and dialysis should be considered.
Benzodiazepines–anxiolytics	Confusion, ataxia, slurred speech	Flumazenil is a benzodiazepine antagonist that is used to reverse the effects of an overdose. Administer flumazenil (0.2 mg) intravenously over 30 seconds and then wait for 30 seconds. Administer it through a large vein to minimize pain at the site of injection. Repeat administration (0.2–0.5 mg) over 30 seconds at 1-minute intervals until the patient responds. Do not exceed 3 mg.
Cannabis	Feeling of well-being, euphoria, altered perception, increased anxiety, paranoia, lack of coordination, increased appetite and thirst, injected conjunctiva tachycardia	Acute anxiety should be treated with benzodiazepines such as lorazepam (1–2 mg), administered orally.
Stimulants (methamphetamine and variants, cocaine)	Hyper-alert state, increased talking, restlessness, elevated temperature, anorexia, nausea, dry mouth, dilated pupils, sweating, neurological seizures, dizziness, paresthesias, hyperactive reflexes, tremor, psychiatric labile affect, insomnia, delirium, aggression, elation, euphoria, hallucinations, agitation, irritability, anxiety, skin picking, cardiac arrhythmias, hypertension, tachycardia	Agitation and psychosis can be treated with haloperidol (5–10 mg) or risperidone (2–4 mg), administered orally. Provide cardiopulmonary support: Stat blood to rule out hypoglycemia. Treat arrhythmias and hypertension, and treat hyperthermia with ice.

(*continued*)

TABLE 2.1 (continued)

Name of the substance	Signs and symptoms	Management
Inhalants: Typewriter-correction fluid, petrol, glues, spray paints, plastic cement, rubber cement, nitrites and nitrous oxide	Symptoms of intoxication include lacrimation, rhinorrhea, salivation, irritation of the mucous membranes, anorexia, vomiting, sleepiness, dizziness, headaches, slurred speech, ataxia, diplopia, euphoria, decreased inhibition, impaired judgment	Agitation and psychosis should be treated with haloperidol (5–10 mg) or risperidone (2–4 mg), administered orally.
Hallucinogen (LSD. MDMA, Mescaline, Psilocybin)	Paranoia, unreliable judgment, anxiety attacks, flashbacks, blissful calm, reduced inhibitions, elation, concentration and motivation, long-term memory loss, especially if there is a latent psychiatric disorder, depersonalization, derealization, fear of losing one's mind, increased blood pressure and heart rate, nausea and vomiting, blurred vision, poor coordination, dilated pupils, sweating	Treatment is aimed at preventing the patient from harming themselves or anyone else. Talking down and support that emphasizes that the bad trip, anxiety, panic attack, or paranoia will pass as the drug wears off is often helpful. Patients are kept in a calm, pleasant, but lighted environment, and are encouraged to move around while being helped to remain oriented to reality. Occasionally, drugs such as lorazepam are given for anxiety. Users may develop dangerously high body temperatures. Reducing the patient's temperature is an essential acute treatment.
Phencyclideine, Ketamine	Anger, irritability, aggression, impaired insight, impaired judgment, nystagmus, hypertension and tachycardia, ataxia, numbness to pain, hyperacusis	Control breathing, circulation, and body temperature. Treating psychiatric symptom: Benzodiazepines, such as lorazepam, are the drugs of choice to control agitation and seizure; haloperidol 2.5–5 mg per day.

BOX 2.3 LABORATORY INVESTIGATIONS

The following is the set of investigations suggested for a patient presenting to the ED with substance abuse:

Complete blood count, blood sugar level, blood urea and creatinine levels, serum electrolytes, liver function tests, test for HIV and VDRL after pre-test counselling, chest X-ray, ECG, ultrasonography of the abdomen and computerized tomography of the brain (to rule out subdural hematoma). Urine toxicology screening can be done and blood alcohol levels assessed depending upon the availability of facilities.

Differential Diagnosis

- Delirium due to other medical causes, e.g. electrolytes disturbance and fever
- Hepatic encephalopathy
- Subdural haematoma

SPECIFIC WITHDRAWAL CONDITIONS

Alcohol Withdrawal

Signs and Symptoms

The following are the signs and symptoms of alcohol withdrawal: Agitation, hyperactivity, anxiety, hallucinations or illusions with clear sensorium, tachycardia, hypertension, tremors, nausea or vomiting, insomnia, tonic–clonic seizures, and increased deep tendon reflexes.

Time Course

The withdrawal symptoms usually begin 4–12 hours after the consumption of alcohol has been stopped or reduced. They are related to a hyper-adrenergic state. The intensity of the symptoms reaches a peak during the second day of abstinence and the symptoms are likely to improve markedly by the fourth or fifth day. In some patients, there is delayed withdrawal, which peaks after three to four days and lasts for eight to ten days. Withdrawal is more severe in the elderly and in malnourished patients, as well as in patients with concurrent medical illness.

Immediate Steps

- *Ensure hydration.* Encourage oral intake of fluids, unless disturbances in consciousness are present. The presence of nausea, vomiting or diarrhea may prevent effective absorption; in such cases, consider intravenous administration of fluids.
- *Correct deficiencies* of electrolytes (sodium, calcium, potassium, and magnesium) by administering fluids intravenously.
- *Consider putting the patient on medication.* For uncomplicated withdrawal, benzodiazepines are the treatment of choice among which, chlorediazepoxide and

lorazepam are the preferred drugs. Depending upon the severity of withdrawal symptoms, the doses can be titrated.

Administer chlordiazepoxide, 25 mg or 50 mg, as required, orally every 6 hours for maximum up to 100–150 mg daily in divided doses. Alternatively, one can administer lorazepam, 2 mg (in those with signs and symptoms of hepatic dysfunction) orally every 2–4 hours for maximum up to 8–10 mg daily in divided doses. The dose should be tapered down and stopped over 7–14 days.

- Propranolol as an adjuvant to benzodiazepines has been shown to be of use in reducing the severity of withdrawal by reducing the hyper-adrenergic state. It should not be prescribed if the heart rate is less than 50. Propranolol at a dose of up to 100 mg should be given to patients with signs of tachycardia and hypertension. Once the pulse rate and blood pressure normalize, propranolol should be tapered by 10–20 mg a day every 3–4 days.
- Thiamine, 100 mg, can be administered intramuscularly twice a day for the first 3–5 days and then orally to complete a course of 7 days. (The first doses should be given intramuscularly because malabsorption is common among alcohol users.) Thiamine is essential to prevent the development of the Wernicke–Korsakoff syndrome, and should be given before initiating parenteral glucose/dextrose saline 1 mg orally every day for 7 days, and vitamin B complex, 1 tablet orally every day for 7 days. Consider magnesium administration (intravenously) 2–4 mEq/kg on day 1 and 0.5–1 mEq/kg daily on days 2–4.

Management of Complications

Seizures: Tonic–clonic convulsions are a complication of alcohol withdrawal among about 5%–15% of patients. They usually develop within 6–48 hours, but can also occur as late as 7 days after the cessation of alcohol use. About 30% of patients who have seizures will develop withdrawal delirium.

Administer diazepam intravenously until the seizure activity ceases. The initial dose should be 5–10 mg. If necessary, this should be repeated at intervals of 10–15 minutes. One can go up to a maximum dose of 30 mg. (Inject slowly, taking at least 1 minute for each 5 mg given.) Lorazepam is a safe alternative for diazepam for the control of seizures.

Anti-epileptics should not be administered unless the patient has a known primary seizure disorder.

Withdrawal delirium (DTs): This is a medical emergency, which occurs in less than 5% of individuals. It usually begins 48–96 hours (or rarely, 1 week) after the cessation of or a decrease in the intake of alcohol. It occurs mostly in individuals who have been drinking heavily for 5–15 years. Withdrawal delirium may last 1–5 days. If the condition is left untreated, the mortality may be as high as 20% (Sellers and Bienenfeld 2001; Kaplan and Sadok 1993).

Alcohol withdrawal delirium is characterized by altered sensorium with disorientation to time, place and person, lapses in memory and judgement, hallucinations and fleeting delusions. In addition to the line of management suggested for simple alcohol withdrawal, the following methods of management are recommended:

- Lorazepam (2 mg) or diazepam (10 mg) may be administered intramuscularly or intravenously if the oral route is not an option. Doses of lorazepam should be repeated till sufficient reduction of the symptoms is achieved. The dose of lorazepam can be repeated at 4–6 hour intervals depending on the level of sedation achieved. A maximum of 14–16 mg of lorazepam can be given in one day. The dose can be titrated in accordance with the level of sedation.
- Haloperidol (2–5 mg) may be administered intramuscularly or intravenously every 2–4 hours to control severe agitation or psychosis. It should be used with caution, however, as it may lower the seizure threshold and is metabolized hepatically.
- If possible, avoid physical restraints as the patient may fight them and cause injury. Specifically, be alert to the possibility of sharp elevations in the creatine phosphokinase level. In extreme cases of delirium and psychosis, physical restraints should be used with care and with the informed written consent of the patient's relative.
- Observe the patient closely for the level of sedation, vital signs, and development of focal neurological signs.
- Put the patient on a high-calorie, high-carbohydrate diet.

Wernicke–Korsakoff syndrome (WKS) is a specific condition generally seen in a patient of long standing alcohol dependence resulting from thiamine deficiency. It is generally agreed that Wernicke encephalopathy results from severe acute deficiency of thiamine (vitamin B1), while Korsakoff psychosis is a chronic neurologic sequela of Wernicke encephalopathy.

Wernicke encephalopathy is characterized by the presence of a triad of symptoms: (i) ocular disturbances (ophthalmoplegia); (ii) changes in mental state (dementia); (iii) unsteady stance and gait (ataxia).

The criteria for the diagnosis of Korsakoff syndrome are (i) anterograde amnesia; and (ii) variable presentation of retrograde amnesia and one of (i) aphasia, (ii) apraxia, (iii) agnosia, a deficit in executive functions.

People with WKS often show confabulation, spontaneous confabulation being seen more frequently than provoked confabulation. Spontaneous confabulations refer to incorrect memories that the patient holds to be true, and may act on, arising spontaneously, without any provocation.

Diagnosis: Diagnosis of WKS is predominantly clinical. MRI brain showing hyperintense signal in the mesial dorsal thalami is a common finding in Wernicke encephalopathy.

Treatment: The onset of Wernicke encephalopathy is considered a medical emergency, and thus thiamine administration should be initiated immediately when the disease is suspected. Prompt administration of thiamine to patients with Wernicke's encephalopathy can prevent the disorder from developing into WKS or reduce its severity.

Patients suffering from Wernicke encephalopathy should be given a minimum dose of 500 mg of thiamine hydrochloride, infused over 30 minutes for 2–3 days. If no response is seen, then treatment should be discontinued; for patients who respond, treatment should be continued with a 250 mg dose delivered intravenously or intramuscularly for 3–5 days unless the patient stops improving. Oral thiamine 100 mg three times a day should be supplemented for 1–3 months to support the recovery process.

Sedative/Hypnotic/Anxiolytic (Withdrawal)

This group of substances includes:

- Benzodiazepines – diazepam, alpraxolam
- Benzodiazepine-like drugs – zolpidem, zaleplon
- Barbiturates and barbiturate-like drugs – phenobarbital, pentobarbital, secobarbital, meprobamate, ethchlorvynol, glutethimide, chloral hydrate, and methaqualone.

Withdrawal symptoms are likely to occur after chronic use of 40–60 mg of diazepam or its equivalents per day, and 400–600 mg of pentobarbital or its equivalents per day.

Signs and Symptoms

The signs and symptoms of withdrawal from these substances are essentially the same as those of alcohol withdrawal.

Time Course

The time of onset and duration of the sedative-hypnotic withdrawal syndrome depend largely on the pharmacokinetics of the particular agent. The initial symptoms may occur within 24 hours of abstinence from the use of a short-acting agent such as pentobarbital, but they may be delayed for as long as one week following abstinence from a longer-acting agent such as phenobarbital.

Immediate Steps

Treatment for benzodiazepine withdrawal includes:

- Shift the patient to equivalent doses of long-acting benzodiazepines, e.g. diazepam, chlordiazepoxide, and clonazepam.
- After the symptoms stabilize, gradually reduce the doses by 20%–30% every third day.
- Psychological interventions may be useful during detoxification from benzodiazepines for the long-term management of anxiety.

Opioid Withdrawal

Signs and Symptoms

In approximate order of appearance, the signs and symptoms of opioid withdrawal are:

- Anxiety, irritability and craving
- Dysphoric mood
- Lacrimation and rhinorrhea
- Insomnia

- Yawning
- Increased sensitivity to pain
- Muscle, bone and joint aches
- Fever (usually low-grade) and hot and cold flushes
- Pupillary dilation, piloerection ("cold turkey") and sweating
- Nausea, vomiting, and diarrhea
- *Hyper-adrenergic stage:* Increased blood pressure, pulse, and respiratory rate
- Muscle twitching and kicking ("kicking the habit").

Time Course

In most individuals who are dependent on short-acting drugs, such as heroin or morphine, the withdrawal symptoms occur within 6–24 hours of the last dose. They peak at 48–72 hours and last 7–10 days. The symptoms may take 36–72 hours to emerge in the case of longer acting drugs, such as methadone or levo-alpha acetyl methadol (LAAM).

Immediate Steps

Opioid withdrawal is uncomfortable, but not life-threatening. The objective of the treatment of withdrawal is to reduce rather than suppress the symptoms. Patients should be told to expect some discomfort, but should be reassured that they will not be allowed to suffer pain. The physician relies on objective findings (e.g. piloerection, sweating, rhinorrhea, papillary changes, tachycardia, and hypertension) to determine whether withdrawal is present; subjective complaints regarding the severity of the withdrawal are less reliable. If the patient is enrolled in a buprenorphine maintenance programme, personnel from the programme should be contacted to verify the daily dosage.

Medication

The main principle of treatment is replacement of the opioid agent. Sublingual buprenorphine has become the replacement of choice in most cases because of its long half-life and the ease with which it can be administered orally. If the patient's daily dosage can be verified through the maintenance programme, this dosage can be safely given to the patient. If not, symptomatic relief can be achieved with 2–4 mg of sublingual buprenorphine in the case of most patients in significant opioid withdrawal. The advantage of such a dosage is that even individuals who have never taken opioids can safely be on this dosage without running the risk of respiratory arrest.

The amount given the first day should be divided into two daily doses on the second day and then tapered at a rate of 10%–20% per day.

Other Complications

Injecting drug users may suffer from certain other medical complications caused by their habit. Be alert to possible signs and effects of endocarditis, trauma, intoxication with other substances, and malnutrition. The possibility of HIV and hepatitis C infection should also be considered.

EMERGENCIES IN SUBSTANCE-INDUCED PSYCHOTIC DISORDERS

Patients presenting with psychosis in the context of substance abuse in emergency settings always pose a diagnostic dilemma to a treating psychiatrist. The clinical presentations closely mimic more serious conditions such as schizophrenia, apart from the history of the substance abuse, which may be difficult to obtain in emergency settings.

The substances generally presenting with substance-induced psychotic disorders include alcohol, cannabis, cocaine, amphetamines, and hallucinogens.

The psychotic disorders occurring during or immediately after substance use are diagnosed as substance-induced psychosis. They are characterized by vivid hallucinations, misidentifications, ideas or delusions of reference or persecution, and psychomotor disturbances in clear sensorium.

For stimulant drugs, such as cocaine and amphetamines, drug-induced psychotic disorders are generally related to high-dose levels or prolonged use of these substances. The diagnosis of substance-induced psychosis is warranted only when the symptoms of psychosis are judged to be in excess of those usually associated with intoxication or withdrawal or severe enough to warrant separate diagnosis. The diagnosis of psychotic state can be further specified by characteristics or specifiers such as predominantly delusional or hallucinatory, schizophrenia-like, and predominantly depressive or manic.

The differential diagnosis includes schizophreniform disorder, schizophrenia, mood disorder with psychotic features, and organic psychosis.

Management

- Patients need to be treated for accompanying intoxication or withdrawal.
- Conduct medical and psychiatric evaluation with special attention to comorbid psychiatric disorders and physical complications due to substance dependence.
- Benzodiazepines such as lorazepam 1–2 mg per orally or intramuscularly every 4–6 hours depending on severity of symptoms. Haloperidol 2–5 mg per orally or intramuscularly can also be used to control the psychosis and agitation.

Legal Aspects

Psychiatric emergencies due to substance abuse pose multiple challenges to the treating physician. These are not only medical and psychiatric, but also legal and ethical. The use of seclusion and restraints remains among the foremost controversial issues in this context (Zitek 2004). The following is a set of guidelines for the use of seclusion and restraints in psychiatric emergencies related to substance abuse.

- Avoid seclusion and restraints, whenever possible.
- Always use seclusion as the first line of management before restraints.
- Seclusion and restraints are warranted only when patients can inflict immediate harm on themselves or others, and should be used for the minimum time possible.
- Take the informed written consent of the patient's relatives before using seclusion or restraints.

Additionally, it must be remembered that many patients may be taking illegal drugs, due to which they may have had a brush with the law or remain at a risk of having a brush with the law. In such cases, full confidentiality must be ensured.

REFERENCES

Benegal, V, Chand, PK and Obot, IS 2009, Packages of care for alcohol use disorders in low- and middle-income countries. *PLoS Med,* 6, e1000170.

Bhalla, A, Datta, S and Chakrabarti, A 2006, A profile of substance abusers using the emergency services in a tertiary care hospital in Sikkim. *Indian J Psychiatry,* 48, 243–247.

Bienenfeld, S and Sellers, MB 2001, Intoxication. In: Bernstein, Ishak, Weiner, Ladds (eds). *On call psychiatry.* 2nd ed. pp. 125–134. Philadelphia: W.B. Saunders.

Gururaj, G, Murthy, P, Girish, N, *et al.* 2011, Alcohol-related harm: Implications for public health and policy in Bangalore, India. Bangalore: NIMHANS, Publication No. 73.

Kaplan, HI and Sadok, BJ 1993, *Pocket handbook of emergency psychiatric medicine: Alcohol withdrawal delirium (DTs).* pp. 104–105. New Delhi: BI Publications.

Saddichha, S, Vibha, P, Saxena, MK and Methuku, M 2010, Behavioral emergencies in India: A population-based epidemiological study. *Soc Psychiatry Psychiatr Epidemiol,* 45, 589–593.

Sellers, MB and Bienenfeld, S 2001, Substance withdrawal. In: Bernstein, Ishak, Weiner, Ladds (eds). *On call psychiatry.* 2nd ed. pp. 135–148. Philadelphia: W.B. Saunders.

Zitek, H 2004, *Emergency psychiatry, legal principles: Seclusion and restraints.* pp. 54–55. New Delhi: Tata McGraw-Hill.

3 Psychotic Disorders including Schizophrenia

Hema Tharoor, T.C. Ramesh Kumar

INTRODUCTION

Psychotic disorders need to be recognized when patients with these present to the emergency department (ED). This chapter outlines the common causes, presentations, and management of this group of disorders. The discussion does not follow any classificatory system – either DSM or ICD, as we believe that the identification and management of these disorders is more important. The chapter thus deals with clinical syndromes and symptoms. In the case of psychosis, the acute emergent presentations often include hallucinations, delusions, speech disorders, and agitation. Psychosis is a symptom or a feature of mental illness typically characterized by radical changes in personality, impaired functioning, and a distorted or non-existent sense of objective reality. Patients arriving in the ED in a psychotic crisis and requiring immediate management may not have been diagnosed with psychiatric illness previously. They often present diagnostic dilemmas in that it may not be clear whether the etiology is organic or psychiatric, and whether they are suffering from a primarily psychotic disorder or a mood disorder. Acute psychosis is classified as a medical emergency requiring immediate and complete attention (Table 3.1). The failure to identify the condition and treat it can result in suicide, homicide, or other types of violence.

SCHIZOPHRENIA

Patients with schizophrenia may be brought to the ED because of behavioral disturbances at the onset or during the course of the illness. Agitation and violence

TABLE 3.1

Mental and Behavioral Disorders Presenting as Acute Psychosis

- Schizophrenia
- Mood disorders – mania/depression
- Brief reactive psychosis
- Substance-induced (alcohol, cannabis)
- Catatonia
- Others, e.g. dementia with psychotic features

occur as prodrome (prior to onset) or as the first episode of psychosis, and indicate relapses during the course of the illness. This requires emergency consultation. While the psychiatric emergency service setting will not be able to provide long-term care for these types of patients, it can provide a brief respite and reconnect the patient to his treating doctor/case manager and/or introduce necessary psychiatric medication. Often, the history obtained in the ED relates to a complication of treatment (adverse effects of a medication) or a crisis arising from socioeconomic factors secondary to schizophrenia (e.g. poverty, homelessness, social isolation, and failure of support systems) (Gerstein and Dyne 2010).

A visit to the ED by a patient suffering from a chronic mental disorder may also indicate the existence of an undiscovered precipitant, such as a change in the lifestyle of the individual or a shifting medical condition. These considerations can play a part in improving the existing treatment plan, if there is one.

MOOD DISORDERS

Mania: Patients with mania are excitable, agitated, impulsive, and violent. Patients in a state of manic excitement come to the ED commonly due to uncontrollable violence or destructive/disinhibited behavior related to mood-congruent grandiose delusions.

Depression: In contrast, patients with severe depression may be suicidal, catatonic (mute), or agitated. They might be brought to the ED following a highly lethal and intentional attempt at self-harm. Young and elderly depressive patients could be in a state of extreme agitation or present with gross self-neglect and refuse treatment. ED presentations among childbearing women include postpartum depression (*see* Chapter 7) characterized by a high risk of suicide or violence.

BRIEF REACTIVE PSYCHOSIS

Hysterical psychosis: This condition, described by Hollander and Hirch (1969), has a sudden and dramatic onset that is temporally related to a profoundly upsetting event or circumstance. Its manifestations include hallucinations, delusions, depersonalization, and grossly unusual behavior. Thought disorders, when they occur, are usually sharply circumscribed and very transient. Affect, if altered, is more volatile than flat. An acute episode seldom lasts longer than 1–3 weeks, and the eruption is sealed off so that there is practically no residue. Hysterical psychosis is encountered most commonly in persons referred to as hysterical characters or personalities when they are faced with trying situations in life or with problems. Indian psychiatrists, such as Wig and Narang (1969), observed that hysterical psychosis in not uncommon in India and opined that hysterical psychosis should be viewed separately from schizophrenia. A retrospective study from south India by Kuruvilla and Sitalakshmi (1982) analyzed the clinical features of hysterical psychosis patients (n=88) and compared them with those of an equal number of persons with catatonic schizophrenia and conversion reaction. The hysterical psychosis patients could be differentiated from patients of hysterical neurosis and schizophrenia. Their long-term prognosis was good and similar attacks did recur in the wake of life stressors.

SUBSTANCE-INDUCED PSYCHOSIS

Most states of intoxication are usually not difficult to diagnose, but intoxications from alcohol, cannabis, cocaine, and amphetamines can mimic the delusions, paranoia, hallucinations, and agitation caused by de-compensated psychotic illnesses. The management of patients in such cases involves the use of benzodiazepines to calm and detoxify them (*see* Chapter 2). In cases of intoxication by pure stimulants and in which there is no underlying psychiatric illness, this is usually sufficient to relieve the symptoms of psychosis benignly. Nicotine deprivation has been found to increase agitation in smokers, especially those with high baseline irritability. Patients with psychiatric illness and substance use disorders smoke at higher rates than the general population, and the incidence of smoking is approximately 70% among patients with schizophrenia (Allen *et al.* 2010). There is a compelling need to improve our recognition of the smoking status of our patients and be more aware of the potential for nicotine withdrawal. The western research finding that nicotine replacement therapy significantly lowered the level of agitation in smokers with schizophrenia in the ED is an eye-opener.

STUPOR AND CATATONIA

Catatonia is a syndrome characterized by the presence of a variety of behavioral and motor symptoms. While individuals with catatonia often cannot provide a coherent history, collateral sources of information, such as their families, might be able to give relevant historical information. The family members can confirm the presence of the typical primary features of catatonia (Table 3.2).

TABLE 3.2

Signs of Catatonia

- Stupor (marked decrease in reactivity to the environment and in spontaneous movements, activity)
- Immobility or withdrawal
- Posturing (voluntary assumption and maintenance of inappropriate or bizarre postures)
- Rigidity (maintenance of a rigid posture against efforts to be moved)
- Staring, grimacing
- Mutism (not talking)
- Negativism (an apparently motiveless resistance to all instructions or attempts to be moved, or movement in the opposite direction)
- Echopraxia/echolalia (meaningless repetition of others' words or actions)
- Waxy flexibility (maintenance of limbs and body in externally imposed positions)

Note: The alternative presentation of catatonia is an excited state possibly with impulsivity, combativeness, and autonomic instability. A history of an excited state should be sought from the family of a person with catatonia, but it is often denied by the family. When present, the episodes of excitement are short-lived and may precipitate collapse due to exhaustion. An excited state of catatonia can be associated with bipolar disorder.

During the initial interview of the patient and the family, elicit a history of possible precipitating events, including infection, trauma, and exposure to toxins and other substances.

- In an emergency setting, the treatable common causes of catatonia must be rapidly considered and ruled out (Table 3.3). It is useful to remember the non-psychiatric causes of catatonia (Table 3.4). Some points to differentiate stupor, whether it is functional or of organic origin, can also help. According to DSM-V criteria, to make a diagnosis of catatonia one has to have a minimum of three of the following twelve clinical features, either observed or elicited during examination: (i) mutism, (ii) stupor, (iii) catalepsy, (iv) waxy flexiblity, (v) agitation, (vi) negativism, (vii) posturing, (viii) mannerisms, (ix) stereotypies, (x) grimacing, (xi) echolalia, or (xii) echopraxia.

The lack of motor and speech abnormalities in delirium helps to differentiate it from catatonia. On the other hand, serotonin syndrome, central nervous system infection, autoimmune encephalopathy or some other medical and neurological conditions encountered in the acute hospital setting may overlap with the signs of catatonia, and in some cases necessitate concomitant treatment for both catatonia and the underlying condition. In the absence of any clinical, physiological, imaging, or other diagnostic markers that are reasonably sensitive and specific in defining catatonia, the diagnosis rests on the clinical history and observation of characteristic signs.

One study found that none of the twelve items that are included in DSM-V possess very high discriminating values for catatonia, but noted that three items (agitation, stereotypies, and mannerisms) had a weak correlation with catatonia. A subsequent study found that stereotypies and mannerisms also have high discriminating values for catatonia (Wijemanne and Jankovic 2015).

STUPOR

In this state the individual appears to be asleep and yet, when vigorously stimulated, may become alert as manifest by eye opening and ocular movement. Other motor activities are limited and there is usually no speech. It may be difficult to differentiate stupor resulting from organic cerebral dysfunction from those with catatonic schizophrenia or

TABLE 3.3

Causes of Catatonia

- Brief reactive psychosis
- Schizophrenia
- Severe depression with catatonic features
- Dissociative states
- Neuroleptic malignant syndrome
- Drugs: 3,4-ethylenedioxymethamphetamine (ecstasy), alcohol, amphetamines, phencyclidine, substance abuse, hypnotic-sedatives

TABLE 3.4

Non-psychiatric Etiologies of Catatonia

- Infections
- Typhoid fever
- Neurocysticercosis
- Viral encephalitis
- Neurosyphilis

- Autoimmune and inflammatory
- Systemic lupus erythymatosis
- Paraneoplastic encephalitis
- Multiple sclerosis

- Cardiovascular
- Takotsubo cardiomyopathy

- Renal
- Renal failure in dementia with Lewy body disease

- Metabolic
- Wilson disease
- Hyponatremia or hypernatremia
- Glucose-6 phosphate deficiency
- Neurodegenerative disorders
- Parkinson disease
- Familial frontotemporal dementia

- Central nervous system
- Posterior reversible encephalopathy
- Subdural hematoma
- Pontine and extrapontine myelinolysis
- Stroke

- Hematology
- Pernicious anemia
- Thrombotic thrombocytopenic purpura

- Medications
- Venlafaxine-associated hyponatremia
- Lorazepam withdrawal
- Paliperidone palmitate
- Dexamethasone
- Zolpidem withdrawal
- Temazepam withdrawal
- Quinolones
- Clozapine withdrawal*
- Manganese neurotoxicity
- Clonazepam/benzodiazepine withdrawal
- Ziprasidone
- Lithium toxicity
- Tramadol and meperidine
- Azithromycin
- Levetiracetam
- Efavirenz

- Surgical causes
- Liver or kidney transplantation
- Temporal lobectomy
- Burns
- Trauma

- Other causes
- Deprivation, abuse, or trauma in pediatric population
- Pregnancy or postpartum

severe depression. The electroencephalogram (EEG) is usually of considerable help as it shows a diffuse abnormality in organic stupor whereas in other forms of stupor it is usually normal. The exception is in patients with catatonic stupor or catatonia. Caloric testing in organic stupor will usually reveal tonic deviation, whereas in psychiatric stupor ocular nystagmus will be present. This is because the fast phase reflects correction following tonic deviation, and this requires the patient to be conscious.

Neurological examination is normal. The catatonic state is characterized by eyes open and unblinking, pupils dilated but reactive, oculocephalic responses absent or impaired, and caloric responses intact. Passive limb movements are met with a "waxy flexibility". This state is difficult to distinguish from organic disease, particularly in lethargic unresponsive individuals. The EEG shows a low voltage fast record rather than the "slowing" of true coma (Cartlidge 2001).

- The emergency physician must quickly consider the presence of neuroleptic malignant syndrome, encephalitis, non-convulsive status epilepticus, and acute psychosis.
  - The physician must find out whether the patient has been exposed to traditional and atypical neuroleptics. While malignant neuroleptic syndrome often follows the initiation of neuroleptic therapy or an increase in the dosage of neuroleptics, the exposure to neuroleptics may be minimal in some susceptible individuals.
  - It must be ascertained whether the patient has had encephalitis. Determine whether there has been a sudden onset of headache, fever, and deterioration in mental functioning.
  - Non-convulsive status epilepticus must be ruled out. Determine whether the patient has a history of seizures and whether he/she has been prescribed anti-epileptic drugs. Find out if EEGs have been performed and if so, review the findings.
  - Acute psychosis must be ruled out. Determine whether the patient has exhibited evidence of delusions and hallucinations. Also, find out if there have been any suicidal or homicidal threats or actions. Record any history of prior psychiatric hospitalization and treatment.
- It is important to ascertain whether there has been a history of similar episodes. Determine whether the events precipitating the current episode are similar to those that precipitated the earlier episode. Record any interventions that relieved catatonia previously.
- Clinicians must identify whether the patient has any comorbid disorders, including schizophrenia, mood disorders, medical conditions, and obstetrical conditions. They should also be alert to the presence of psychological stressors.
- Catatonia has occurred in patients after treatment with levetiracetam and levofloxacin.

The individual's predominant level of activity is either markedly slow or extremely high. The patient's behavior may shift suddenly and unpredictably from one state to the other.

- In the excited state, people with catatonia may injure themselves and assault others. They may also experience autonomic instability manifested as hyperthermia, tachycardia, and hypertension. Individuals in the excited state are at a risk of collapsing due to exhaustion.
- In the immobile state, the individual may not move. Akinesia and stupor are synonyms for this state. The patient may appear unresponsive to external stimuli. He/she may be unable to eat, and may die unless parenteral nutrition and fluids are administered. People with catatonia may exhibit catalepsy, the persistent maintenance of spontaneous or imposed postures.

INVESTIGATIONS

- It is necessary to take a complete blood count and carry out chemical analyses of the blood. In particular, hyponatremia and other metabolic abnormalities must be ruled out.
- Elevations of serum creatine kinase and white blood cell counts, and abnormal liver

function test results are common laboratory findings in catatonia. It is important to immediately measure the serum creatine kinase level, take the white blood cell count, and perform liver function tests to rule out neuroleptic malignant syndrome.
- The level of serum ceruloplasmin should be determined to rule out Wilson disease.
- Encephalitis must be ruled out.
- The CT scan of a person with catatonia may reveal increased ventricle-to-brain ratios. However, CT scans cannot be used to establish the diagnosis of catatonia. The main value of CT scans for patients with catatonia is to rule out other treatable disorders, such as normal pressure hydrocephalous.

MANAGEMENT

Treatable conditions must be identified immediately. Specifically, neuroleptic malignant syndrome, encephalitis, non-convulsive status epilepticus, and acute psychosis must be diagnosed and treated. Neuroleptic malignant syndrome, encephalitis, and non-convulsive status epilepticus constitute neurological emergencies that merit admission to a neurological or medical intensive care unit (Brasic, Benbadis and Catatonia 2010).

Acute psychosis merits admission for intensive psychiatric inpatient evaluation and treatment.

- The use of traditional neuroleptics is avoided because of the possible development of neuroleptic malignant syndrome.
- Successful treatment of catatonia has been reported with several medications, including lorazepam, clonazepam, dantrolene, and olanzapine.
- When non-convulsive status epilepticus, diffuse encephalopathy, and other neurological disorders have been ruled out, electroconvulsive therapy (ECT) is indicated for patients who do not respond to pharmacotherapy in five days or who exhibit malignant catatonia. ECT is effective for many patients with catatonia, including those with catatonia secondary to mood disorders, autistic disorder, and other pervasive developmental disorders. ECT is beneficial for patients with catatonic schizophrenia. The onset of catatonia merits hospitalization so that the work-up may be done and an intervention can be provided for assaultiveness. Refusal to eat requires parenteral nutrition. Autonomic instability requires the administration of intravenous fluids and monitoring of the vital signs.

PSYCHOSIS AND EMERGENCIES IN SPECIAL POPULATION GROUPS

THE ELDERLY

Elderly persons in a state of psychiatric emergency form a small percentage of all elderly patients treated in EDs. However, it is difficult to accurately diagnose and understand behavioral emergencies among the elderly. Emergency behavioral syndromes in the elderly include confusion, agitation, psychosis, and behavioral regression. The causes of these syndromes in the elderly include delirium, dementia, side-effects of medication, physical illnesses, depression, and alcohol intoxication/dependency (Tueth 1994). The management of the elderly is discussed in Chapter 15.

Children

The majority of children/adolescents displaying "psychotic" behavior are likely to be delirious because of drug-induced states, and sometimes, physical illness such as cerebral tumors, lobar pneumonia, encephalitis, seizures, and electrolyte abnormalities.

Drug-induced states, especially those caused by the use of belladonna derivatives and amphetamine-like drugs, and chronic use of marijuana may mimic psychosis. However, psychosis is possible if there are no signs/symptoms suggestive of physical illness, the young person's behavior is highly disturbed and he/she is postpubertal.

Schizophrenia

The main symptoms are hallucinations (usually auditory), delusions, disorganized speech and behavior, and decline in general function. Young people often have a "florid" presentation characterized by highly disturbed behavior, including agitation and extremely bizarre ideas (sometimes bodily symptoms), which may compel them to seek medical help.

Bipolar Disorder

Teenagers who are manic are overactive, and have poor sleep, racing thoughts, and grandiose ideas. They may display disinhibited behavior, and often have auditory hallucinations, and delusions. Many teenagers who are manic are also very irritable, becoming angry when questioned, and occasionally aggressive. Teenagers with a depressive illness have depressive symptoms, but may also have delusions with depressive themes. People may dismiss both the manic and depressive states as "adolescent turmoil".

Other Psychotic Disorders

Children and adolescents may develop other psychotic disorders, such as delusional disorders, but these are rare.

Management in Children

It is necessary to take a detailed medical history and make a thorough assessment (including drug screens).

- Children with schizophrenia and bipolar disorder need skilled psychiatric care (often inpatient) and medication. Therefore, refer anyone you suspect to be suffering from schizophrenia or a manic episode to a psychiatrist. Urgent assessment is necessary.
- In a psychiatric emergency (such as refusal by a seriously suicidal person to get admitted or exhibiting dangerous aggressive behavior), commitment under the Mental Health Act might be required.
- If you have immediate concerns regarding the safety of a patient, it is legally possible to restrain him or prevent him from leaving the hospital. However, psychiatric services must be contacted as soon as possible, if this proves necessary.

PSYCHOSIS IN MENTAL RETARDATION AND DEVELOPMENTAL DISABILITIES (MR/DD)

Patients of normal intellect who have schizophrenia display psychiatric, cognitive, and neurological problems, as well as psychosocial dysfunction. The application of the diagnostic criteria of psychosis to moderate or severely retarded individuals creates immediate problems because many subjects have poor psychosocial function in addition to their impaired cognition. Significant numbers of patients with schizophrenia have borderline intellectual function. A patient with schizophrenia and "low IQ" may present initially to the mental retardation clinic. On the other hand, some patients with schizophrenia may actually suffer from compromised intelligence.

Management

The assessment of psychosis in non-verbal patients requires behavioral observation. Patients may respond to non-existent stimuli by becoming agitated or displaying self-injurious behavior (SIB), such as banging their head in response to auditory hallucinations. The abrupt onset of psychotic symptoms in the mentally retarded person should suggest delirium or other mental problems, and substance abuse in the mildly retarded individual. Psychotic symptoms can occur in the setting of depression and mania; however, these individuals generally exhibit symptoms of mood disorder prior to the onset of psychotic symptoms. In an older person with mental retardation, psychosis can occur in the form of dementia. Some of these patients who also have epilepsy run a greater risk of developing psychotic symptoms and individuals with temporal lobe seizures run the greatest risk of developing schizophrenia-like syndromes. Psychotic symptoms often worsen behavioral problems, e.g. SIB and aggression. The therapeutic aim of antipsychotics is to reduce the symptoms described by the patient and caregiver or the symptoms as measured by behavioral monitoring. Mildly retarded patients can describe symptomatic changes produced by medications or behavioral interventions. The clinician must depend on behavioral symptoms to determine the efficacy of medication in the case of severely retarded persons.

CULTURE-BOUND SYNDROMES – EMERGENCY PSYCHOSIS?

Latah Betul

Latah betul, "real latah" or "true latah", a phenomenon found to occur in Malaysia, is characterized by the apparent loss of control over behavior and by echolalia, echopraxia, and automatic obedience. The histories of persons with latah betul suggest that in some individuals, extreme stress may precipitate the onset of the disorder. The reports published on latah betul suggest a diagnosis of catatonia.

Amok (or Mata Elap)

This syndrome has been found to occur most frequently among Malayan natives, but has also been reported in other cultures. It consists of a dissociative episode, preceded by a period of introspective brooding and followed by an abrupt onset of unprovoked and uncontrolled rage (an outburst of violent, aggressive, or homicidal behavior). In the latter stage, the affected persons may run about savagely attacking objects and killing people or animals in their way. The rage is directed indiscriminately at everybody or anything in the vicinity. The episode of amok tends to be precipitated by a perceived insult or slight and seems to be prevalent only among males. The episode of amok is often accompanied by persecutory ideas, automatism, and amnesia for the period of the episode. It is followed by exhaustion and a return to the premorbid state.

Instances of amok may occur among individuals with pre-existing psychotic disorders, during a brief psychotic episode, or may represent the onset or exacerbation of a chronic psychotic process.

SPIRITUAL EMERGENCE AND EMERGENCY

"It is a far, far better thing to have a firm anchor in nonsense than to put out on the troubled seas of thought." – J.K. Galbraith

Spiritual emergence has been defined as "the movement of an individual to a more expanded way of being that involves enhanced emotional and psychosomatic health, greater freedom of personal choices, and a sense of deeper connection with other people, nature, and the cosmos" (Spiritual emergency or emergence). An important part of this process is an increasing awareness of the spiritual dimension in one's life and in the universal scheme of things. When spiritual emergence is rapid and dramatic, the process can become a crisis, and spiritual emergence becomes spiritual emergency. This has also been called transpersonal crisis, acute psychosis with a positive outcome and positive disintegration. It may take the form of non-ordinary states of consciousness and may involve unusual thoughts, intense emotions, visions, and other sensory changes, as well as various physical manifestations. The episodes often revolve around spiritual themes or social issues such as migration.

Management

Comprehensive social, psychiatric, biological, racial, and cultural assessments are required. Those with delusional possession require antipsychotics and non-pharmacological treatments. Traditional, culturally sanctioned mechanisms of resolving distress are likely to be unsuccessful in the case of patients who have delusional possession states, but may be helpful for those with dissociative disorders. The greatest difficulty lies in distinguishing the dissociative group from those with suggestibility states. Therefore, the assessment of suggestibility, ritualizing, and dissociative states requires consultation with those who have expertise in the religious/spiritual, cultural, racial and sociological aspects of a particular possession state. Members of the community to which the patient belongs should be consulted at all stages of the assessment and treatment process.

CONCLUSION

It is a common misconception that there are no real emergencies in psychiatry. This chapter has highlighted the common psychiatric emergencies and described their management. As for schizophrenia, the variability in symptom expression, diagnostic requirement of chronicity, and lack of pathognomonic features makes diagnosis of this condition in the ED only provisional at best. As a diagnosis-by-exclusion, schizophrenia must be distinguished from the numerous psychiatric and organic disorders that can also lead to psychotic disturbances in thinking and behavior. However, the best teacher is experience, and if one is still unclear about the diagnosis or management, it would be wise to consult a senior consultant before any treatment initiation.

REFERENCES

Allen, MH, Debanné, M, Lazignac, C, Adam, E, Dickinson, LM and Damsa, C 2011, Effect of nicotine replacement therapy on agitation in smokers with schizophrenia: A double-blind, randomized, placebo-controlled study. *Am J Psychiatry,* 168, 395–399.

Brasic, JR and Benbadis, SR. Catatonia – follow-up. Available at emedicine.medscape.com/article/1154851-overview (accessed on 8 October 2010).

Cartlidge, N 2001, States related or confused with coma. *J Neurol Neurosurg Psychiatry,* 71 (suppl I), i18–i19.

Gerstein, PS and Dyne, PL. Schizophrenia in emergency medicine. Available at http://emedicine.medscape.com/article/805988-overview emedicine.medscape.com/ article/805988-overview (acceessed on 18 May 2010).

Hirsch, SJ and Hollender, MH 1969, Hysterical psychosis: Clarification of the concept. *Am J Psychiatry,* 125, 81.

Kuruvilla, K and Sitalakshmi, N 1982, Hysterical psychosis. *Indian J Psychiatry,* 24, 352–359.

Spiritual emergency or emergence. Available at http://easternhealingarts.com/Articles/SpititualEmergency.html

Tueth, MJ 1994, Diagnosing psychiatric emergencies in the elderly. *Am J Emergency Medicine,* 12, 364–369.

Wig, NN and Narang, RL 1969, Hysterical psychosis. *Indian J Psychiatry,* 11, 93.

Wijemanne, S and Jankovic, J 2015, Movement disorders in catatonia. *J Neurol Neurosurg Psychiatry,* 86, 825–832.

4 Psychiatric Emergencies in Grief

Hema Tharoor, R. Padmavati

"There are things that we don't want to happen but have to accept, things we don't want to know, but have to learn, and people we can't live without but have to let go."

– Author unknown

INTRODUCTION

Grieving the death of a loved one has an ancient history. From time immemorial, cultures have provided the bereaved with advice and rituals to address, and express, the experience of grief (Aries 1981). The terms "bereavement" and "grief" are used inconsistently in the literature to refer to either the state of having lost someone to death, or the response to such a loss.

Historically (Zisook 1995), the early understanding of loss crystallized from Freud's description of the work of grief as a "painful relinquishing of ties from the deceased". Recently, theorists, influenced by the "attachment theory" have emphasized that the work of grief involves attachment as much as separation. The attachment theory speaks of a human instinct to form strong, persistent affectional bonds. A natural response to the loss of an attachment bond is separation anxiety, which generates an intense and predictable behavior aimed at recouping or reviving the lost relationship.

Researchers have suggested that the word bereavement be used to refer to the fact of the loss; the word grief should then be used to describe the emotional, cognitive, functional, and behavioral responses to the death. Also, grief is often used more broadly to refer to the response to other kinds of loss. For example, people grieve the loss of their youth, of opportunities, and of functional abilities. The word mourning is sometimes used interchangeably with bereavement and grief, usually referring more specifically to the behavioral manifestations of grief, which are influenced by social and cultural rituals, such as funerals, visitations, or other customs. Complicated grief, sometimes referred to as unresolved or traumatic grief, is the current designation for a syndrome of prolonged and intense grief that is associated with substantial impairment in work, health, and social functioning.

PHENOMENOLOGY OF GRIEF

The process of grieving does not follow a strict pattern. The different phases of grieving can be described as an overlapping and fluid process that is dependent on various factors, such as the survivors' personality, their previous life experiences, their past psychological history, the significance of the loss, the relationship with the deceased person, the survivor's social network, health and other resources, and intercurrent of life events (Box 4.1). There is ample evidence to indicate that the bereavement process does not end within a prescribed interval; some aspects persist indefinitely.

The phenomenology of grief needs to be understood because the overt manifestations of underlying grief in the emergency room may range from severe depression, panic attacks, dissociative states to suicide attempts.

BOX 4.1 PHASES OF GRIEF

1. Shock and denial (minutes, days, weeks)
   - Disbelief and numbness
   - Searching behaviors
2. Acute anguish (weeks, months)
   - Waves of somatic distress
   - Withdrawal
   - Preoccupation
   - Anger
   - Guilt
   - Restlessness, agitation
   - Amotivation, aimlessness
   - Identification with the bereaved
3. Resolution (months, years)
   - Return to work
   - Resumption of old roles
   - Assumption of new roles
   - Re-experiencing of pleasure

ACUTE GRIEF REACTION

This occurs in the early aftermath of a death. The reaction can be intensely painful and is often characterized by behaviors and emotions that would be considered unusual in normal everyday life. These include intense sadness and crying, other unfamiliar dysphoric emotions, preoccupation with thoughts and memories of the deceased person, disturbed sleep and appetite, difficulty concentrating, and a relative lack of interest in other people and the activities of daily life (apart from the role the person plays in mourning the deceased). This form of grief is to be distinguished from a later form of grief, i.e. integrated or abiding grief, in which the deceased is easily called to mind, often with associated sadness and longing.

INTEGRATED GRIEF

During the transition from acute to integrated grief, which usually begins within the first few months of the death, the wounds begin to heal and the bereaved person finds his or her way back to a fulfilling life. The reality and meaning of the death are assimilated and the bereaved is able to once again engage in pleasurable and satisfying relationships and activities. Even though the grief has been integrated, the individuals do not forget the person they lost. Nor do they cease to feel sad or stop missing the loved ones. The loss becomes integrated into autobiographical memory and the thoughts and memories of the deceased are no longer preoccupying or disabling. Unlike acute grief, integrated grief does not preoccupy the mind persistently or disrupt other activities.

However, there may be periods when the acute grief reawakens. This can occur at the time of significant events, such as holidays, birthdays, anniversaries, another loss, or a particularly stressful time.

COMPLICATED GRIEF

Complicated grief, a syndrome that occurs in about 10% of bereaved people, results from a failure to make the transition from acute to integrated grief. Psychiatric and medical interventions are required because of the increased morbidity and risk of suicide associated with complicated grief (Devan 1993).

Bereaved individuals suffering from complicated grief find themselves in a repetitive loop of intense yearning and longing that becomes the major focus of their lives. The yearning is accompanied by inevitable sadness, frustration, and anxiety. People suffering from complicated grief have been found to be at increased risk for cancer, cardiac disease, hypertension, substance abuse, and suicidality.

Among bereaved spouses over the age of 50 years, 57% of those suffering from complicated grief had suicidal ideation compared to the remaining 24% who did not endorse suicidal thoughts (Szanto, Shear and Houck 2006). Among adolescent friends of adolescent suicides, young adults with complicated grief were 4.12 times more likely to endorse suicidal thoughts than subjects who did not have syndromal level complicated (Prigerson, Bridge and Maciejewski 1999). In studies of clinical populations, complicated grief was associated with a high rate of suicidal ideation, a history of suicide attempts and indirect suicidal behavior, not explained by co-occurring major depression, and with elevated rates of lifetime suicide attempts in the case of bipolar patients (Simon, Pollack and Fischmann 2005). Once established, complicated grief tends to be chronic and unremitting. Clearly, it must be taken seriously and treated appropriately.

PATHOLOGICAL GRIEF

The term "pathological grief" is sometimes applied to people who are unable to work through their grief despite the passage of time. A pathological grief reaction may be diagnosed if a long time (one or more years) has passed and the grieving person is not improving. Such patients may present with chronic depression or mummification (preservation of all the personal belongings of the dead one). The patient may report sensing the presence of the deceased person or hearing his or her voice. The patient may also suffer from a sense of guilt regarding the commission or omission of acts in relation to the death. When the family doctor labels someone's grief as pathological, he or she is indicating that the resolution of the grieving process is delayed and that professional help is needed. The use of the term does not imply any disrespect towards the patient.

There is no absolute time-frame within which grief is considered pathological, although there are cultural norms that serve as guidelines. In both the West and the East, a person might be judged as being "stuck" if the individual is still actively grieving 18–24 months after the loss. An unremitting "overly intense" grief process of shorter duration might also be labeled pathological. If we adopt these ideas as guidelines, it is important to encourage people who appear to be stuck in the grief process to seek professional grief counseling.

ACUTE GRIEF REACTIONS IN THE ELDERLY

The elderly accumulate losses suddenly, in rapid succession, with agonizing repetition, and in great volume. People in mourning are usually offered sympathy, care, and attention by others. However, the elderly may entirely miss out on such opportunities that allow one to mourn in a healthy way since grief reactions among them often follow the so-called "devious patterns of grief". In other words, the grief reactions are disguised by clusters of other symptoms. These reactions may appear to be physical ailments, anxiety syndromes, major depression, and even senile dementia. Due to the misleading reactions, the practitioner's evaluation and approach to treatment are often misdirected and the underlying etiology of grief remains undetected. Another reason why a proper diagnosis is not made is the ironic fact that the elderly are often expected to simply "grin and bear" their losses due to their significant longevity. Many families and practitioners believe that grieving is not relevant to the aged. The fact that the elderly respond to loss instinctively like any other person rather than in the context of their old age goes largely unappreciated. As losses accrue with age, the person begins to increasingly value his remaining attachments and gives them up only begrudgingly. Seemingly nondescript personal objects generate intense emotions in the elderly when a loss occurs, since these objects may serve as surrogate relatives and are potent reminders of previously lost important people.

GRIEF REACTIONS IN CHILDREN AND ADOLESCENTS

Children and adolescents present to the emergency department (ED) only in case of uncontrollable agitation, crying, a dissociative state, a suicide attempt, or intoxication (alcohol) in reaction to the loss.

The significance of grief and bereavement in adolescents and children is underappreciated by families and clinicians. The loss can range from the death of a parent, grandparents, siblings, friends, or pets to other significant people in their lives. The reactions to the loss depend on the child's age. A toddler or a child in preschool asks the same question again and again, needing reassurance. Older children understand death more completely, although they might not be able to perceive of the finality or permanence of death. The timetable for grieving is different from that in the case of adults and is unpredictable. The manifestations of grieving are variable. Children are often seen to be playing and laughing in the midst of grieving adults. On the other hand, they often cry uncontrollably at an unrelated sight, or experience a fresh and intensified fear of death and dying. More than any other age group, grieving adolescents display denial, anger, and reckless behaviors.

ANTICIPATORY GRIEF

Anticipatory grief is a term that describes the grief process a person undergoes before a loss actually occurs. Clayton *et al.* (1973) attempted to define anticipatory grief in the context of subjects whose spouses had short terminal illnesses (six months or less), those whose spouses had longer terminal illnesses (more than six months), and those whose spouses died suddenly (in less than five days). Gilliland and Fleming (1998) conceptualized anticipatory grief as a multidimensional phenomenon similar to grief. They empirically compared and contrasted the features of anticipatory grief and conventional grief, and addressed the effects of anticipatory grief on post-death bereavement. It was found that the anticipatory grief experienced by the spouses of terminally ill persons was marked by more intense levels of acute symptomatology than was conventional grief. Furthermore, it was found that anticipatory grieving played a role in helping the individual to adapt. Those experiencing anticipatory grief tended to have less intense and acute levels of symptoms during post-death bereavement.

DISTINGUISHING BETWEEN GRIEF REACTIONS AND MAJOR DEPRESSION

Bereavement evokes depressive symptoms. The DSM-IV has made efforts to demarcate a normal grief reaction from major depression.

Bereavement	Major Depression
Symptoms may meet syndromal criteria for major depression, but survivor rarely has morbid feelings of guilt and worthlessness, suicidal ideation, or psychomotor retardation	Criteria as described in DSM-IV
Dysphoria often triggered by thoughts or reminders of the deceased	Dysphoria often autonomous and independent of thoughts or reminders of the deceased
Onset within first two months of bereavement	Onset can be any time
Duration of less than two months	Can become chronic, intermittent, or episodic
Functional impairment transient and mild	Clinically significant distress or impairment

MANAGEMENT

Most of the support that people receive after a loss comes from friends and family. Doctors and nurses may also be a source of support. The approach to supporting a person in grief should be based on common sense.

Crisis intervention

The various forms of grief can present as a crisis or escalate into one and force patients to consult emergency services. Patients can come to the ED in a state of acute anxiety or dissociation (pseudoseizures), with major depression or with suicidal feelings, depending on the extent and type of grief. Appropriate intervention during the crisis has a significant effect on the grief response and the subsequent resolution of the loss (Holland and Rogich 1980). It is mandatory to determine the phase of grief and decide on supportive treatment accordingly.

Supportive treatment usually entails:

- Accepting the wide range of responses of the bereaved as "normal reactions"
- Using appropriate words in order to console the bereaved
- Facilitating grieving instead of restricting the release of emotions
- Setting a limit on extreme reactions, such as self-destructive behaviors and aggression.

Pharmacotherapy

Most persons grieving a loss are usually greatly distressed during the period immediately following the loss. However, a great majority recover during the following weeks. Therefore, clinicians are reluctant to utilize pharmacotherapy during the immediate aftermath.

The use of medications may be necessary when the bereaved person is extremely agitated or psychotic. In the emergency room, short-acting benzodiazepines (e.g. lorazepam) or high-potency neuroleptics (e.g. haloperidol) may prove effective. Atypical antipsychotics at low/optimum doses may also be useful and necessary in cases of pathological grief presenting as psychosis. Pharmacological treatment (antidepressants) may also be warranted in the first month after the trauma as some survivors may experience extreme and persistent arousal in the form of anxiety, panic, hypervigilance, irritability, and insomnia.

It is necessary to remember that drug therapy should be combined with counseling and other forms of non-pharmacological interventions.

Suicide Risk Assessment

Suicidal ideations or attempts at suicide have been reported by patients of all age groups. The presence and extent of suicidal tendencies depend on the patient's perceived sense of loss. Suicide risk assessment (*see* Chapter 8) is of critical importance and needs to be carried out in all phases of grief.

Grief Counseling

After the patient has been stabilized in the ED, he should be recommended for grief counseling, depending on the type and nature of the loss (Box 4.2).

Family Work

As bereavement affects all the family members of the deceased, it is essential to extend the intervention to all family members after the acute crisis has been resolved.

EFFICACY OF GRIEF THERAPY

Meta-analyses of the grief literature for children and adults suggest that the long-standing assumption that grief therapy is appropriate for all grievers is no longer tenable (Mancini, Griffin and Bonanno 2012). Grief therapy is better suited for children and adults with marked and persistent distress following a loss. Further, grief treatments

BOX 4.2 PRINCIPLES OF GRIEF COUNSELING THAT NEED TO BE ADHERED TO DURING THE MANAGEMENT PROCESS

- Work in the context of the family
- Respect religion, culture of the bereaved
- Empathy without over-identification
- Detachment
- Therapeutic neutrality
- Ensure conditions to allow verbal expression of grief
- Listening to feelings behind the spoken words
- Help bereaved develop new activities, interests

targeted to distressed grievers are efficacious, but less so than general psychotherapy (Wampold 2001). The reasons for the smaller effect sizes of grief treatments remain unclear. Several explanations have been given in the literature; a few are given below.

One, grief treatments expose a subset of grievers to iatrogenic effects, reducing the overall efficacy. In their review of grief treatments, Jordan and Neimeyer (2003) cited an unpublished meta-analysis in which 38% of grievers showed deterioration following treatment. Although this assertion has been debated on statistical and methodological grounds (Wampold 2001; Currier, Holland and Neimeyer 2010), there is a growing consensus that grief treatments should be reserved for persons with marked and persistent levels of grief-related distress.

Two, grief treatments include persons whose symptoms would resolve on their own, limiting the differences between intervention and control conditions. Evidence suggests that bereaved persons typically show some improvement across time, regardless of whether they receive treatment (Bonanno and Lilienfeld 2008).

This perspective is reinforced by three prototypical trajectories that characterize people's reactions to loss (Currier, Neimeyer and Berman 2008). About 50% are resilient and cope remarkably well with loss and would obviously not require professional intervention. A subset of grievers (10%–20%) show a more traditional pattern of acute grief symptoms followed by more gradual recovery. Clinical interventions are most suitable when there is a pattern of prolonged (or chronic) grief (10%–15%) in which elevated symptoms may grow worse and persist for years following the loss. The failure to target treatment specifically to persons whose grief reactions will not resolve on their own (prolonged grievers) may be another reason for the relatively lower levels of efficacy of grief treatments.

Finally, earlier grief treatments were based on outmoded theories about loss. In a recent meta-analysis of cognitive behavioral therapy (CBT) and other grief therapies, Currier *et al.* (2010) reported that CBT was superior to other therapy types in direct comparisons. However, when investigator allegiance, a crucial confounding factor, was controlled, these differences were no longer significant, and CBT was no more efficacious than comparison treatments. Thus, improvements in treatment approach have not as yet provided an explanation for the lower level of benefit observed in grief treatments.

REFERENCES

Aries, P 1981, *The hour of our death*. pp. 614. Oxford: Oxford University Press.

Bonanno, GA and Lilienfeld, SO 2008, Let's be realistic: When grief counseling is effective and when it's not. *Prof Psychol Res Pract,* 39, 377–378.

Clayton, PJ, Halikas, JA, Maurice, WL and Robins, E 1973, Anticipatory grief and widowhood. *Br J Psychiatry,* 122, 47–51.

Currier, JM, Holland, JM and Neimeyer, RA 2010, Do CBT-based interventions alleviate distress following bereavement? A review of the current evidence. *Int J Cogn Ther,* 3, 77–93.

Currier, JM, Neimeyer, RA and Berman, JS 2008, The effectiveness of psychotherapeutic interventions for bereaved persons: A comprehensive quantitative review. *Psychol Bull,* 134, 648–661.

Devan, GS 1993, Management of grief. *Singapore Med J,* 34, 445–448.

Gilliland, G and Fleming, S 1998, A comparison of spousal anticipatory grief and conventional grief. *Death Studies,* 22, 541–570.

Holland, L and Rogich, LE 1980, Dealing with grief in the emergency room. *Health Soc Work,* 5, 12–17.

Jordan, JR and Neimeyer, RA 2003, Does grief counseling work? *Death Studies,* 27, 765–786.

Mancini, A, Griffin, P and Bonanno, G 2012, Recent trends in the treatment of prolonged grief. *Curr Opin Psychiatry,* 25, 46–51.

Prigerson, HG, Bridge, J and Maciejewski, PK 1999, Influence of traumatic grief on suicidal ideation among young adults. *Am J Psychiatry,* 156, 1994–1995.

Simon, NM, Pollack, MH and Fischmann, D 2005, Complicated grief and its correlates in patients with bipolar disorder. *J Clin Psychiatry,* 66, 1105–1110.

Szanto, K, Shear, MK and Houck, PR 2006, Indirect self-destructive behavior and overt suicidality in patients with complicated grief. *J Clin Psychiatry,* 67, 233–239.

Wampold, BE 2001, *The great psychotherapy debate: Models, methods, and findings*. New York: Routledge.

Zisook, S 1995, Death, dying and bereavement. In: Kaplan, HI and Saddock, BJ (eds). *Comprehensive textbook of psychiatry*. 6th ed. pp. 1713–1728. New York: Williams and Wilkins.

5 Emergency Treatment of the Acutely Disturbed and Aggressive Patient

Lopa Winters, Julian Eaton

INTRODUCTION

Agitated and violent behavior has long been associated with mental illness in the public domain. This association is largely driven by stigma and misconception. It is important to remember that people with mental illnesses are far more often the victims of, rather than the perpetrators of violence, and the wrongly held belief that they are dangerous has been used to justify unnecessary incarceration and human rights abuse, sometimes on a systematic and officially sanctioned scale, and sometimes in an informal but pernicious way at the level of communities. Challenging these popular but false beliefs and promoting care and support based on the principle of "least restrictive practice" is an essential component of service development.

Sometimes, however, disturbed and occasionally violent behavior can occur in clinical settings, and studies have shown that aggression is a feature of 10% of psychiatric emergencies (most commonly associated with psychosis or substance misuse). Preparedness for such a situation thus needs to be a part of clinical training and practice (Huf, Coutinho and Adama 2007). An appropriate and sensitive approach to these challenging situations will make it more likely that patients are able to receive care that maintains their dignity and autonomy, diffuse the immediate risks, and potentially improve long-term outcomes. The possibility of encountering hostile, uncooperative, or violent patients is often one of the greatest causes for anxiety among clinicians, but if they are trained and equipped to manage such situations in a safe, calm, and psychologically containing manner, it can significantly reduce their anxiety, as well as the risk of injury. The aim is to ensure that the person becomes calm enough to engage with, so that a mutually agreed treatment process can move forward.

It is a reality of psychiatric care that there are certain times when patients (especially psychotic patients) do not want to receive treatment, even when most people would accept that it is in their best interest because their behavior is posing a threat to themselves, to others, or to property. They may not accept treatment because the symptoms of their disorder make them irritable or aggressive, they may have false beliefs (delusions)which make them fear that those around them are trying to harm them, or they may not believe that they are sick ("lack insight").

Medical ethics and international standards such as the United Nations Conventions on the Rights of Persons with Disabilities dictate that a patient has the right to autonomy in making decisions about their own care. Only when the right of the patient to consent to treatment is in conflict with other principles, such as the right of others not to be harmed, do many national legal frameworks allow clinicians to (temporarily) act against a person's wishes, usually in what is assumed to be their "best interest". Many countries have codified in law the circumstances under which this may happen. Usually this involves a combination of medical professionals and legal representatives defining the conditions under which a person is judged to lack the capacity to understand the situation, or the possible consequences of their actions. Any intervention must be shown to be proportionate, accepted by a body of professions to be of benefit to the patient in their condition, and temporary, being given against the person's will only until they have mental capacity to make autonomous decisions again. It is worth noting that there is considerable dispute over whether professionals should ever be allowed to adopt the role of making decisions for patients in their "best interest", i.e. a patient always retains legal capacity even when judged to have a compromised mental capacity. One of the consequences of a paternalistic view about the perceived lack of capacity of people with mental illness has been long-term containment in institutions, still common in many countries. In many cases, insufficient efforts are made to seek the patient's view prior to acting on their behalf, which is perhaps an inevitable result of the power imbalance in these circumstances. Various means of supportive decision-making, use of advocates, or asking the person's wishes in advance should play a more prominent role in managing these circumstances.

In many countries, such principles of best practice are either not established in law or not universally understood. It is therefore necessary for medical and social professionals to be particularly careful about protecting human rights in the course of their work. They are often in a position to exert a positive influence at times of great difficulty for patients and their families, and are respected enough by society to ensure that people with mental illnesses are treated with dignity even when they are at their most vulnerable (Box 5.1).

The most important thing is preparation. Institutions and organizations delivering mental healthcare should have good practice guidelines for the management of

BOX 5.1

Treatment should never be given against a person's will unless they are likely to pose a serious risk to themselves or others, if they do not receive treatment. In most cases, if sufficient skill and time are used, it is possible to find a solution that is acceptable to all parties.

Remember that it is against a person's human rights to force them to take treatment against their will, and forcing treatment will only make them suspicious of the care you might provide them in the future.

emergencies, and should ensure that their staff is adequately prepared for emergencies. For individuals at risk of presenting acutely in a disturbed way, it is possible to discuss with them in advance what their preferred means of management might be. This will ensure not only that considered decisions are taken with respect to human rights, but also that any treatment is appropriate and safely given.

STEP-BY-STEP APPROACH TO ASSESSMENT AND MANAGEMENT

Here, we outline an approach to managing disturbed and aggressive behavior in people with mental illness. The emphasis is on the safety of all concerned, respect for the rights of the person involved, and promotion of engagement with the person and their family throughout what is often a distressing situation (*see* Flowchart 5.1).

Safety First!

The risks can be reduced significantly by attempting to obtain as much information as possible before having to act.

- Ask the family, referrer, etc. about the potential risk when taking the referral or planning a visit.
- Find out if the person is known to suffer from mental illness.
- Find out if the person is known to abuse any substance and when they last used anything.
- Ascertain if the patient is suffering from persecutory ideation ("paranoid"). Find out the nature of any paranoid beliefs he may have so that you can attempt to allay his fears.
- Find out if the patient has access to potential weapons.
- Find out if the patient has been violent or aggressive in the past. Past violent behavior is known to be the best predictor of future behavior.
- Identify ways of leaving quickly, if necessary. When you are in an enclosed space, always place yourself nearer to the exit than to the patient.
- Make sure that there are sufficient people available to help ensure your safety in case of violence. Determine whether it is necessary for the police to be involved.
- Ensure that you yourself are not carrying sharp implements, jewellery, neckties, or objects that can potentially be used by the patient to harm themselves or others.

Share: Collaboration and Consent Come First

- Engaging the patients as much as possible is of paramount importance. Try to talk to the patients directly rather than just to those around them, no matter how distracted they seem.
- Even the most apparently aggressive and hostile patients respond well to "talking down" approaches, and feeling that their views and wishes are being taken seriously.
- Remember that patients may behave in a hostile and aggressive manner when they themselves feel vulnerable, threatened, and attacked in some way. Make sure they feel understood.
- Respectful engagement is important for the future therapeutic alliance, which may

Flowchart 5.1: Emergency Treatment of Aggressive Patients

Preparation is essential for the safe management of a person who is behaving in an aggressive or violent way. The people involved should know what to do in advance, and not just react to the emergency in an unpredictable manner.

The first thing to do is to assess the situation. The following 4 S's must be kept in mind.

Safety first
- Ensure that you and others are not at risk.
- Ensure that the patient does not have access to any weapons.
- Find out about any history of previous violence.

Share
- Engage and build a rapport with the patient as far as possible.
- Talk calmly to the patient and avoid confrontation.
- As far as possible, ensure that the patient is able to make decisions about the treatment.

Step back (physically)
- Do not encroach on the patient.
- Speak in a calm, slow, and steady manner. Be reassuring, not confrontational and accusing.

Step back (mentally)
- Find out from the patient's family/community what provoked the situation.
- Assess if the person has symptoms of mental illness, such as delusions or thought disorder, which might be prompting the behavior.
- Find out if the patient has been drinking alcohol or using drugs.
- Ascertain whether a physical condition, such as delirium or pain, could be causing the behavior.

Steps in management

1. Use non-pharmacological techniques such as "talking down" to diffuse the situation

If this does not succeed after a while or if the situation is escalating: ↓

2. If the person is mentally ill (not just angry or intoxicated), and it is felt that drugs are needed, try to persuade the person to take oral medication.

If the patient refuses oral medication and is still in need of sedation: ↓

3. Administer rapid tranquilization.

Before administering rapid tranquilization, the team needs to be prepared.
- The drugs should be prepared by the person who will be injecting them.
- There should be at least two people to hold one limb each, and another person to administer the prepared injection – a minimum of five people. One person should give the instructions to the rest of the team.
- Once the person has been sedated, he should be routinely monitored.

Make plans for the future: ↓

A single treatment will not solve the problem beyond the immediate situation. The patient must make regular visits, and a long-term treatment plan for the coming months must be made with the patient and their family. If they do not continue to come for reviews, they should be followed up in the community.

be a very long-term one. Patients often remember the initial interactions after the situation has been resolved.

- A patient's experience in the initial encounter is likely to affect his future compliance with drugs.
- A collaborative approach is of vital importance. The clinician must always attempt to adopt such an approach as it makes the situation safer, as well as less traumatic for the patient and his family even if medications are administered eventually.

Step Back (Physically)

- When faced with a disturbed patient, it is important to maintain a distance that is both safe for you and non-threatening to the patient.
- Patients with persecutory ideas may perceive of encroachment upon their personal space as a form of confrontation or attack and may lash out in self-defense.
- Keep at arm's length from the patient.
- Do not touch the patient as they may misinterpret the gesture, even if it was intended to be empathetic.
- Do not stare at the patient as this may be considered confrontational.
- Speak in a calm, slow, and steady manner. Be reassuring, not confrontational and accusing.

Step Back (Mentally)

Think about how the circumstances might affect the patient's behavior and whether you can modify them for the better.

- When a patient is acutely disturbed, they and those around them are fearful and anxious.
- You may be the only one at the time to be in a position to view the situation with "a fresh pair of eyes" and a clear mind, so take the time to step back mentally, and think and assess the situation objectively.
- Try to determine what appeared to trigger the disturbed behavior, or make it worse.
- Make an attempt to ascertain whether the agitation, irritability, or aggression is related to mental illness or not.
- Give some thought to whether the patient's condition could be secondary to pain, physical illness, a social problem, or any other problem, even if combined with an underlying mental illness.
- Remember that even if a patient has a diagnosis of mental illness, they may be agitated for reasons other than psychosis or delusional beliefs.
- Consider whether there are any factors you can address to resolve the situation. This might include promising to look into issues troubling the patient after the immediate situation has been resolved.

Non-pharmacological Approaches First

Try "talking down". Encourage the patient to talk about their concerns and listen attentively. Try to address them if possible, and find alternative solutions to confrontation.

- Even the most apparently aggressive patients often collaborate if you devote time to them, remain calm, and listen.
- Reduce any tension in the environment by removing anyone whose presence is counterproductive, anyone who does not have a relevant role to play (bystanders), and generally minimize the number of people involved. It may help, for example if in a very public or unsafe place, to suggest moving somewhere more appropriate, if possible.
- It is important to respect the patient's wishes and human rights. Even in the difficult situation you are confronted with, it is often possible to obtain the client's consent and proceed with treatment.
- Insist that the purpose of treatment is to improve the situation for the patient first (even when others may want to punish or harm the patient) and take care to avoid unnecessary treatment involving restriction which might be abusive.

Pharmacological Management

When all alternative methods have been explored, it may be necessary to use medication to prevent the patient from posing a further risk of injury to themselves or others.

Background

The use of drugs to bring about sedation in an acutely disturbed patient is referred to as "rapid tranquilization" or "RT". One can use a number of agents, such as antipsychotics, benzodiazepines, and antihistamines, alone or in combination (Alexander 2004). The use of an antipsychotic drug when there is evidence of psychosis has the advantage that it amounts to initiating treatment, but it is important to recognize that a single dose is not sufficient and long-term treatment will be necessary. Long-term treatment should include providing appropriate psychosocial care; advising the patient and his family on the need to avoid precipitating factors, particularly drugs such as cannabis, if it is a factor involved; and prescribing appropriate medication to avoid relapses, if the patient is diagnosed with chronic psychosis.

Different medication is available in different places, and hospitals or community services may have different policies or traditions. Worldwide, guidelines are often influenced by local practice, and there is limited evidence to argue that one regimen is universally the most appropriate. Here, we present some different treatment options. It is essential that before the need to administer emergency treatment arises, any service should decide which treatment option its staff should use. It should also ensure that the staff is trained to administer the treatment. Further, the necessary equipment and drugs should be available.

Rapid tranquilization guidelines in the UK and the USA recommend the oral or intramuscular administration of lorazepam, often combined with haloperidol (National Institute for Health and Care Excellence, Clinical Guidelines 2015).

Many high-income countries are increasingly using atypical antipsychotics such as olanzapine as they are said to be "calming" rather than sedating, but such medications are expensive or unavailable in some low-income countries. In general, there is little evidence published on the most appropriate approaches to use in low-income countries (Huf, Coutinho and Adama 2007; Alexander 2004; Taylor, Paton and Kerwin 2005–06).

Haloperidol alone or a combination of haloperidol and lorazepam is commonly used in low- and middle-income countries such as India and Brazil (Huf, Coutinho and Adama 2007). A common practice in these countries is to add promethazine, a sedative antihistamine with anticholinergic properties, to haloperidol to accelerate the onset of sedation and minimize the adverse effects of antipsychotics, such as acute dystonic reactions (Huf, Coutinho and Adama 2007). Haloperidol and promethazine are both on the WHO's list of essential drugs (Raveendran *et al.* 2007).

Benzodiazepines alone, such as intramuscular lorazepam, 4 mg, have been shown to be as effective as haloperidol, 10 mg, plus promethazine, 25 mg or 50 mg; however, if rapid sedation is required, the latter is superior to benzodiazepines alone (Alexander 2004). There is good reason to administer an antipsychotic in combination with a benzodiazepine if there is evidence of psychosis and the patient is very disturbed.

	Medication and dose*	**Notes**
Choice 1	Lorazepam, 4 mg, PO or IM	Effective, particularly when there is no clear evidence of psychosis
Choice 2	Olanzapine, 10 mg, PO or IM	To be given for psychosis, where available
Choice 3	Haloperidol, 10 mg, with promethazine, 25–50 mg, PO or IM	Best choice for rapid effect in psychosis
Choice 4	Haloperidol, 10 mg, IM or PO with diazepam, 5–10 mg, PO	If other benzodiazepines are not available, diazepam should not be given IM. Beware of the risk of dystonic reaction.

PO oral IM intramuscular

* These doses are for a healthy adult of average build. Seek advice of an experienced doctor or pharmacist when treating other groups as treatment options or doses may need to be adjusted.

Best practice guidelines have changed significantly in recent decades, but a recent study in Africa showed that prescription patterns had changed minimally and most psychiatrists continued to prescribe chlorpromazine and diazepam, as according to them, prescribing habits were more likely to be influenced by the availability of these drugs than by cost or preference (Bawo 2011). Some bad practices remain in use, including the intramuscular administration of diazepam (which is unpredictably absorbed by this route), rather than the oral administration of diazepam or other benzodiazepines. The lack of availability of intramuscular anticholinergic medications for use in cases of acute dystonic reactions is also a problem in some countries.

Intramuscular paraldehyde should no longer be used as it is painful, and more humane and effective options exist.

Offer oral medication to the patient. Remember that the medication being given to the patient is for the treatment of mental illness, and not for punishment. It might happen that the patient becomes so sedated as to sleep, but this is not the aim of intervention (National Institute for Health and Care Excellence, Clinical Guidelines 2015).

- Oral treatment is just as effective as injections. If medical treatment is necessary, it is much better if oral or injected medication is given with the patient's consent.
- Keep explaining to the patients that you have their best interest in mind, and that giving them medication is not a punishment. Tell them that threatening or dangerous behavior is not acceptable and that they need treatment for their own good.
- Explain to the patient that you want to seek their consent to give them treatment.
- If the patient does not consent, and the situation is judged to require treatment without their consent, explain this to them.

Rapid Tranquilization

If all efforts to calm the patient down have failed, and they are judged to need medication but refuse to take it, then rapid tranquilization should be considered.

Before Administering Rapid Tranquilization (Box 5.2)

- Ask yourself, "Have I exhausted all other possibilities?"
- Ascertain whether the patient has had the drug before and if they suffered any side-effect.
- Make sure the drug you will use has not expired and has been prepared for administration.
- Try to persuade the patient to accept an oral dose first or to consent to intramuscular treatment.
- If it is necessary to treat the patient without their consent, ensure that you explain what you are about to do before you do it, particularly making it clear that it is not a punishment.
- Explain why you are giving the drug and what it will do.
- Ensure that there are enough people at hand to help you administer the drug safely, particularly to hold the patient still if they struggle. If a patient is very disturbed, five people will be required.
- Make sure the team is prepared in advance and each person knows their role. One person (usually the senior clinician) should have the role of coordinating the administration of the medication in a well-organized and calm manner.

BOX 5.2

Rapid tranquilization can be extremely traumatic psychologically for the patient and their family. It is not without serious risks and adverse effects, including heart and breathing problems. Therefore, the decision to administer rapid tranquilization must not be taken lightly and all other possibilities must be explored first. The risks are higher among children (who should not be given rapid tranquilization), the elderly, and pregnant women, as well as those with significant heart disease, dementia, or epilepsy. Doses of medication suggested in this chapter may need to be adjusted for these groups.

BOX 5.3

If the patient has a dystonic reaction (painful muscle spasms, such as flexing of the neck to one side and rolling of the eyes) or other side-effects, such as rigid muscles, anticholinergic medication, such as procyclidine or benzhexol, should be used to treat the problem.

- In order to be able to do the job safely and quickly, the person administering the medication should not need to worry about holding the patient still.
- The helpers should be warned not to obstruct the patient's airway or hurt them while holding them.
- Try to maintain a calm environment and preserve the patient's dignity while they are being held until sedated.

After-care: Patient

- Emphasize the importance of regular monitoring (e.g. every 15 minutes for the first hour and every 30 minutes after that) to check the patient's breathing, mental state, and side-effects of medication (Box 5.3).
- Tell the patient and caregivers about the side-effects that may occur and what they can do about these.
- Make a plan for the long-term care of the patient and support of the family. Set a date for the first review.
- Arrange a meeting with the patient to discuss their experience of rapid tranquilization. This will help to engage them and make them more amenable to treatment.
- Consider making a joint contract with the patient with respect to any future episodes in which rapid tranquilization may be necessary. Though this may not be legally binding, it helps empower the patient and makes them feel that they are involved in their own care.
- Note whether any serious adverse effects have been mentioned in the patient's case notes and share these with the team.

After-care: Clinical Team

- Managing acutely disturbed patients can provoke anxiety and be unpleasant for the clinicians involved, so it is important to arrange for a meeting with peers or supervisors to share experiences, develop knowledge and skills, and promote reflective learning.
- Ensure that the learning from experiences is integrated into policy development and training so that practice improves with time.

CONCLUSION

Preparation for emergency treatment is a necessary precaution, given that there are occasions when such treatment will be necessary in a mental health service. It is essential that staff should be aware both of the ethical considerations and the medical options for dealing with aggression when it occurs. Of primary importance is to preserve a patient's dignity and autonomy as much as possible, while following a methodical process, which ensures that any necessary treatment is given in the least restrictive way that preserves dignity. This in turn will ensure the best long-term outcome for the patient.

REFERENCES

Alexander, J, Tharyan, P, Adams, C, John, T, Mol, C and Philip, J 2004, Rapid tranquilization of violent or agitated patients in a psychiatric emergency setting. *Br J Psychiatry,* 185, 63–69.

Bawo, J 2011, Rapid tranquilization agents for severe behavioural disturbance: A survey of African psychiatrists' prescription patterns. *Tropical Doctor,* 4, 49–50.

Huf, G, Coutinho, ESF and Adama, CE 2007, Rapid tranquilisation in psychiatric emergency settings in Brazil: Pragmatic RCT of intramuscular haloperidol versus intramuscular haloperidol plus promethazine. *Br Med J,* 335, 869.

National Institute for Health and Care Excellence, Clinical guidelines 2015, Violence and aggression: Short-term management in mental health, health and community settings. Available at https://www.nice.org.uk/guidance/published?type=cg&title=violence.

Raveendran, NS, Tharyan, P, Alexander, J, Adams, CE and TREC-India II Collaborative Group 2007, Rapid tranquilization in psychiatric emergency settings in India: Pragmatic RCT of intramuscular olanzapine versus intramuscular haloperidol plus promethazine. *BMJ,* 335, 865.

Taylor, D, Paton, C and Kerwin, R 2005–06, *Maudsley prescribing guidelines*. 8th ed. Abingdon: Taylor and Francis.

6 Psychiatric Emergencies Associated with Drug Overdose

S. Haque Nizamie, Sai Krishna Tikka, Nishant Goyal

The essential features of an emergency are urgency, severity, its unscheduled nature, lack of previous adequate assessment or planning, and ensuing indecisiveness and conflict. A psychiatric emergency is defined as a severe disturbance of behavior, mood, or thought that needs immediate attention; it refers to acute symptoms and psychological and/or physical distress, which are beyond the patient's coping capacity at the time (Antai-Otong 2001). The tense and chaotic atmosphere in a psychiatric emergency, the time constraints, the transient doctor–patient relationship, and the lack of confidence and faith of the patient's relatives in psychiatrists make a psychiatric emergency different from the usual psychiatric contacts (Jena 1999). Drug overdosage is one such chaotic situation. It is included in the broad rubric of adverse drug events. It occurs when a person takes more than the medically recommended dose of a particular drug. When a person takes an overdose of a drug, the side-effects of that drug become more pronounced. Further, the person may also experience other effects that would not occur with normal use. Drug overdosage can be a consequence of accidental overuse, intentional/deliberate misuse, or iatrogenic errors.

Drug overdosage can be related to psychiatry in a variety of circumstances. A psychiatrist might be called for an opinion on the neuropsychiatric symptoms presented by drug overdose patients. A drug overdose patient might present primarily to a psychiatrist. A patient might have used one or more psychotropic drugs for intentional overdose, or a psychiatrist might be called to assess and manage patients who have taken an overdose of drugs in a bid to commit suicide. This chapter deals with the assessment and management of each of these circumstances.

DRUG OVERDOSE IN MEDICAL SETTING: PSYCHIATRIC SIGNS AND SYMPTOMS

A clinician dealing with psychiatric emergencies related to drug overdose must have a good idea of the psychiatric manifestations of overdose of various drugs, whether clinically prescribed (Table 6.1) or clinically not prescribed/poisons (Table 6.2), and

TABLE 6.1

Various Clinically Prescribed Drugs and Psychiatric Manifestations of their Overdose

Drug	Psychiatric signs and symptoms	
Acetaminophen	Early/ acute Massive doses rarely cause changes in mental status. Late/ chronic Encephalopathy	
Amantadine	Early/ acute Agitation, visual hallucinations, nightmares, disorientation, delirium slurred speech, ataxia, myoclonus, tremors, and sometimes seizures; also neuroleptic malignant syndrome	
Amphetamines	Early/ acute Euphoria, talkativeness, anxiety, restlessness, agitation, seizures, coma Late/ chronic Stereotypical behavior (such as picking at the skin), paranoia, and paranoid psychosis; psychiatric disturbances may persist for days or weeks	
Antiarrhythmic drugs: Tocainide and mexiletine	Early/ acute Sedation, confusion, coma, seizures	
Anticholinergics	Early/ acute Delirium (part of anticholinergic syndrome)	
Anticonvulsants	Gabapentin	Early/ acute Somnolence, slurred speech
Anticonvulsants	Lamotrigine, levetiracetam	Early/ acute Drowsiness, lethargy
	Tiagabine	Early/ acute Somnolence, confusion, agitation, depression
	Topiramate	Early/ acute Sedation, confusion, slurred speech, anxiety
	Vigabatrin	Early/ acute Sedation, confusion, agitation, delirium, psychosis (hallucinations, delusions)
	Zonisamide	Early/ acute Somnolence, agitation
Anti-herpes drugs	Acyclovir	Early/ acute Hallucinations and confusion after IV administration

(*continued*)

TABLE 6.1 (*continued*)

Drug	Psychiatric signs and symptoms	
Anti-herpes drugs	Vidarabine	Early/ acute Confusion, hallucinations, psychosis
Antipsychotics	Early/ acute Neuroleptic malignant syndrome	
Baclofen	Early/ acute Hallucinations and seizures with abrupt withdrawal	
Bromides	Late/ chronic Bromism – restlessness, irritability, ataxia, confusion, hallucinations, psychosis, weakness, stupor, coma	
Calcium channel blockers	Early/ acute Stupor, confusion	
Colchicine	Early/ acute Delirium, seizures, or coma	
Dextromethorphan	Early/ acute Restlessness, visual, and auditory hallucinations Serotonin syndrome	
Ergotamine	Early/ acute Psychosis, seizures, and coma occur rarely	
Mefloquine	Early/ acute Dizziness, vertigo, hallucinations, psychosis, seizures	
Non-nucleoside reverse transcriptase inhibitor (NNRTI): Efavirenz	Early/ acute Confusion, disengagement, dizziness, hallucinations, insomnia, somnolence, vivid dreams	
Thyroid hormone	Early/ acute Headache, anxiety, agitation, psychosis, confusion	

Source: Adapted from "Specific poisons and drugs: Diagnosis and treatment", 2004, In: Olson, K.R. (ed). *Poisoning and drug overdose*. 4th ed. pp. 66–404. New York: Lange Medical Books/ McGraw-Hill

dietary supplements (Table 6.3). Psychiatric manifestations can be caused either by acute ingestion of a drug in excessive dose or excess accumulation of a drug due to the long-term and chronic use of the drug. Altered mental status, seizures, psychosis, and agitation are the commonest presentations of drug overdose. All these generally occur as acute effects. The other psychiatric manifestations reported are emotional changes such as euphoria and anxiety, as observed in the case of amphetamine overdose; speech disturbances such as becoming over-talkative, again as observed in the case of amphetamine overdose, and slurred speech, as seen in the case of gabapentin overdose; and sleep disturbances, including nightmares, as seen in the case of amantadine and

TABLE 6.2

Various Non-prescribed Drugs/Poisonous Substances and Psychiatric Manifestations of their Overdose

Drug	Psychiatric signs and symptoms
Arsenic	Early/ acute Lethargy, agitation, or delirium
Boric acid, borates, and boron	Early/ acute Hyperactivity, agitation
Carbon disulfide	Early/ acute – short-term (days to weeks) Mood change, frank delirium, psychosis
Carbon monoxide	Late/ chronic Persistent vegetative state, subtler personality, and memory disorders (among survivors of serious poisoning)
Chlorinated hydrocarbon pesticides (Lindane, etc.)	Early/ acute Confusion, tremors, obtundation, coma, seizures
Gamma-hydroxybutyrate (GHB)	Early/ acute Withdrawal symptoms include tremors, paranoia, agitation, confusion, delirium, visual, and auditory hallucinations
Isopropyl alcohol	Early/ acute Mimics drunkenness from ethanol, with slurred speech, ataxia, stupor
Manganese	Late/ chronic Atypical psychosis mimicking schizophrenia (chronic low dose)
Mercury Especially elemental (metallic) mercury – Hg^o vapour and organic (alkyl) mercury	Early/ acute Fatigue, insomnia, anorexia, and memory loss; there may be an insidious change in mood to shyness, withdrawal, and depression
Nerve agents: GA (Tabun), GB (Sarin), GD (Soman), GF and VX	Late/ chronic Neuropsychiatric changes as sequelae
Nitroprusside (cyanide)	Late/ chronic Hyperventilation, anxiety, agitation, seizures
Organophosphorus and carbamate compounds	Early/ acute Agitation, seizures, coma
Phosphorus	Early/ acute Headache, delirium, seizures, coma

(continued)

TABLE 6.2 (*continued*)

Drug	Psychiatric signs and symptoms
Polychlorinated biphenyls (PCBs)	Early/ acute Neurobehavioral changes in newborns and children
Selenium	Early/ acute Rapid deterioration of mental status with restlessness progressing to coma

Source: Adapted from "Specific poisons and drugs: Diagnosis and treatment", 2004, In: Olson, K.R. (ed). *Poisoning and drug overdose*. 4th ed. pp. 66–404. New York: Lange Medical Books/ McGraw-Hill

TABLE 6.3

Various Dietary Supplements and Psychiatric Manifestations of their Overdose

Dietary supplements and alternative remedies	Anabolic steroids, used for body-building	Early/ acute Aggressiveness, mania or psychosis
	Mahuang (ingredient: various Ephedra spp.), used for enhancement of athletic performance and to suppress appetite	Early/ acute Insomnia, psychosis, seizures
	Yohimbine, supposedly an aphrodisiac	Early/ acute hallucinations
Vitamin A	Late/ chronic Headache, altered mental status, blurred vision due to increased intracranial pressure	
Vitamin D	Late/ chronic Altered mental status	

Source: Adapted from "Specific poisons and drugs: Diagnosis and treatment", 2004, In: Olson, K.R. (ed). *Poisoning and drug overdose*. 4th ed. pp. 66–404. New York: Lange Medical Books/ McGraw-Hill

efavirenz overdose. Overdose due to the chronic use of a drug is by and large relatively rare, and there are only a few drugs that cause such overdose. Bromism, chronic overdose of bromides, was at one time responsible for 5%–10% of admissions to psychiatric facilities because it causes frank psychosis. Certain interesting and some of the rarest manifestations are associated with chronic drug overdose, for example, carbon monoxide overdose may cause subtle personality disorder; amphetamine chronic overdose is associated with stereotypical behavior in the form of skin-picking;

and nitroprusside overdose may cause hyperventilation (Tables 6.1 and 6.2). Late or chronic overdose of caffeine is termed caffeinism, which is characterized by nervousness, irritability, anxiety, tremulousness, twitching of muscles, insomnia, and palpitations. Table 6.3 presents the psychiatric manifestations of overdose of dietary supplements such as anabolic steroids and vitamins.

Apart from anabolic steroids, an overdose of steroids used in clinical medical settings is also known to cause psychiatric manifestations. The reported incidence of steroid psychosis is 3%–57% (Ling, Perry and Tsuang 1981; Lewis and Smith 1983). The risk factors for steroid psychosis are female sex, doses of above 40 mg/day in the case of prednisolone, and long-term administration (Ling, Perry and Tsuang 1981; Hall *et al.* 1979). Steroid psychosis occurs within the first two weeks of corticosteroid therapy and is dose-related (Brown, Khan and Nejtek 1999). The psychiatric manifestations are often both affective, in the form of over-talkativeness, distractibility, or low mood, and non-affective, in the form of hallucinations or core delusions. It is, however, depression that is the most prevalent among these patients, its incidence being as high as about 40% (Ling, Perry and Tsuang 1981; Hall *et al.* 1979). The treatment involves a reduction in the dose or discontinuation of steroids. The use of psychotropic agents becomes essential in such a setting because a reduction in the dose or discontinuation of the steroid results in worsening of the underlying disease requiring steroid therapy. Antipsychotics are the mainstay of treatment, while lithium has been used to treat mood symptoms, both manic as well as depressive (Sicgal 1978). Tricyclic and tetracyclic antidepressants should be used cautiously as they have been reported to induce the exacerbation of agitation (Hall, Popkin and Kirkpatrick 1978).

Antitubercular Drugs

Discussion on the psychiatric manifestations caused by an overdose of antitubercular drugs acquires particular significance in the context of developing countries. With increase in the number of treatment-seekers for tuberculosis, the number of patients presenting as psychiatric emergencies due to overdose of a certain drug in the antitubercular treatment regimen also tends to rise. Most antitubercular drug-associated psychoses have been reported to be caused by isoniazid (Prasad, Garg and Verma 2008). The following may be the psychiatric manifestations of an isoniazid overdose:

- *Psychosis:* excessive argumentation, restlessness, agitation, and irritability, or euphoria, emotional instability, grandiose ideas, and even complex delusions
- Obsessive–compulsive neurosis
- Mania (Alao and Yolles 1998).

The duration of the psychotic symptoms varies widely, from one week to four months (Prasad, Garg and Verma 2008). Isoniazid is believed to produce psychiatric manifestations by causing vitamin B6 deficiency, as well as by inhibiting the activity of brain pyridoxal-5-phosphate, which, in turn, leads to a decrease in brain gamma-aminobutyric acid and other synaptic transmitters (Prasad, Garg and Verma 2008). Therefore, pyridoxine is known to be effective in prevention as well as treatment of isoniazid psychosis (Sievers and Herrier 1975; Snider 1980). However, psychosis that is non-responsive to pyridoxine has been reported (Chan 1999), and this requires treatment with antipsychotics.

Overdose of another antitubercular drug, rifampicin, is also known to cause toxic psychosis (Salafia and Candida 1992). Only rare instances of ethambutol-related psychosis have been reported. The symptomatology is similar to that of isoniazid psychosis and the mechanism is not known (Prasad, Garg and Verma 2008). An overdose of cycloserine, too, causes excitement, anxiety, aggression, confusion, depression, suicidal ideation, and psychosis, along with seizures (Lawrence Flick Memorial Tuberculosis Clinic 1998).

Second-line antitubercular drugs, such as ciprofloxacin, have been reported to cause psychiatric manifestations. Ciprofloxacin overdose can cause restlessness, anxiety, agitation, and disorientation, along with visual and auditory hallucinations, two days after the initiation of treatment, but the symptoms last for less than 48 hours (Norra *et al.* 2003). An acute overdose of antitubercular drugs responds well to activated charcoal, if given early, and hemodialysis.

Antimalarials

Chloroquine and mefloquine are the common antimalarial drugs that can cause psychiatric manifestations. Chloroquine is the drug of choice for prophylaxis as well as treatment of uncomplicated malaria. An acute overdose of this drug is exceedingly dangerous. A dosage as small as 1 g can be fatal for children, while in the case of adults, a dosage of 6 g can be fatal (Bhatia and Malik 1995). The emergency psychiatric manifestations caused by an overdose of chloroquine are convulsions and psychosis. These occur between 2 and 40 days of the initiation of treatment and may last from 2 days to 8 weeks (Bhatia and Malik 1995). Chloroquine can induce psychosis at doses ranging from 1–6 g (Bhatia and Malik 1995). Most commonly, the patient suffers from an affective psychosis. Mania due to a chloroquine overdose is treated with antipsychotics such as olanzapine as long as the patient is symptomatic (Vacheron-Trystram *et al.* 2004).

Mefloquine, used in the treatment of chloroquine-resistant Plasmodium falciparum malaria, has side-effects such as dizziness, insomnia, vivid dreams, nightmares, and light-headedness. Psychosis due to an overdose of mefloquine, though rare, is a psychiatric emergency. The general incidence of severe neuropsychiatric manifestations has been estimated to be about 1 in 215 therapeutic users or 1 in 10,000–15,000 prophylactic users (Weinke *et al.* 1991). Even though there are reports of psychotic symptoms persisting for a long time (Potasman, Berry and Seligmann 2000), the psychosis generally resolves when the drug is discontinued. The use of atypical antipsychotics, such as risperidone, has been shown to be effective, with the psychosis resolving within a few days (Kukoyi and Carney 2003). Mefloquine-induced panic attack is another rare entity. The patient may present to a psychiatric emergency set-up. Only nine such panic attacks were described in an observational study of 16,491 subjects on mefloquine prophylaxis (Meier, Wilcock and Jick 2004). Other quinine derivatives such as hydroxychloroquine (Ward, Walter-Ryan and Shehi 1985) and quinacrine hydrochloride (Evans, Khalid and Kinney 1984), as well as quinine itself (Jerramand Greenhalgh 1988; Verghese 1988), have been reported to cause psychosis. A newer antimalarial alpha/beta arte ether has also been reported to cause manic symptoms among Indian adolescents, compelling them to visit the psychiatric emergency (Haq *et al.* 2009).

MANAGEMENT OF COMMON SYMPTOMS OF DRUG OVERDOSE IN MEDICAL SETTING

The protocol for the management of all drug overdoses is more or less similar – diagnosis of the overdose and assessment of the drug of which the overdose has been taken, followed by management of the Airway, Breathing, and Circulation, and Decontamination and enhanced Elimination (ABCDE of stabilization). Antidotes for the particular drug are used, provided they are available and compatible. Emergencies related to drug overdoses constitute a unique type of psychiatric emergency, in which maintaining the airway, breathing, and circulation are an important step (Walker 1983).

Altered Mental Status

Among the various signs and symptoms associated with overdosage, the most common and serious psychiatric presentation is altered mental status, which includes declining levels of consciousness such as confusion, stupor, and coma. Most likely, the altered mental status is caused by depression of the central nervous system, especially that of the reticular activating system. Another reason might be cerebral infarction or intracranial bleeding caused by the particular drug. Altered mental status may also be related to post-drug-induced seizure phenomenon. If such a possibility exists, it is necessary to perform a CT scan of the brain. The treatment is initiated after ruling out other causes, such as electrolyte imbalance, hypoglycemia, and encephalitis or meningitis. The treatment mainly involves maintaining the airway, breathing, and circulation, which includes oxygen supplementation. Specific measures include providing dextrose (until hypoglycemia is ruled out), thiamine (to alcoholics and patients with vitamin deficiencies to prevent Wernicke syndrome), and naloxone (if respiratory depression is observed) (Olson 2004).

Seizures

Another common neuropsychiatric presentation of drug overdosage is seizures. Seizures may be single and brief or multiple and sustained. Drug-induced seizures or seizures caused by an electrolyte imbalance or withdrawal from alcohol or a sedative-hypnotic drug are likely to be primary generalized, while those caused by focal mechanisms are likely to be partial seizures with secondary generalization. Idiopathic epilepsy has to be ruled out by taking the patient's past and family history to ascertain the presence of seizure disorder. As in the case of altered mental status, the treatment of seizures starts with maintaining the airway, breathing, and circulation. Naloxone may be administered if the cause of the seizures is hypoxia resulting from associated respiratory depression. Anticonvulsants should be started according to the routine protocol for seizures, but have to be administered slowly as these can cause hypotension and cardiac or respiratory arrest. The literature provides evidence supporting the use of diazepam, lorazepam, midazolam, phenobarbital, pentobarbital, and propofol (Olson 2004).

Agitation and Psychosis

The most common psychiatric symptoms of drug overdose are agitation and psychosis. Psychosis includes delusions, especially paranoid, hallucinations, especially visual, and also catatonia, which may occur in those who have taken a phencyclidine overdose. The most crucial element of the assessment of these symptoms of drug overdose is the differentiation of these symptoms from those of a functional psychotic disorder or a metabolic disturbance. Clarity of sensorium and the predominance of auditory modality hallucinations are a hallmark of functional psychosis. Electrolyte screening and neuroimaging are required to rule out metabolic, focal infectious, and an oncological origin of these symptoms. Adequate sedation with the help of benzodiazepines and antipsychotic support with drugs such as haloperidol are the specific modes of treatment for this category of symptoms (Olson 2004).

Violence

This is where the safety of the clinicians and staff becomes the primary consideration. The assessment of patients who have become violent as a result of drug overdose includes identification of certain manifestations in patients. In the context of drug overdoses, the following types of patients are more likely to become violent than others (Walker 1983):

- Patients experiencing drug intoxication or withdrawal, especially with amphetamines, phencyclidine, and alcohol
- Delirious patients
- Postictal patients (ictus secondary to drug overdose)
- Patients with electrolyte disturbances secondary to overdose
- Depressed patients
- Males
- Those belonging to the lower social classes
- Those with a history of fire-setting or other impulse control disorders.

The violence might also be secondary to psychosis or result from anger at being rescued from an intentional overdosage (suicide attempt).

A search for weapons with a metal detector should be a standard practice when the patient enters the emergency department. The interviewer should have access to an exit that ensures that the interviewer does not have to walk past the patient, and the interview room should not have any objects that can be used as a weapon by the patient. The clinician should maintain a body buffer zone of approximately 2 meters. Wearing a white coat/identification batch is helpful. Various non-verbal and direct measures can help to calm the patient. The methods of self-protection include non-verbal manoevers such as keeping still, being calm and humble, shaking hands, and showing interest by leaning forward. The direct manoevers include telling the patient to sit down, talking in a reassuring way, ringing the alarm bell or calling for help, picking up a potential weapon, and managing to run or fight back. If the patient fails to respond to verbal interventions, restraints should be applied. As far as drug therapy is concerned, non-specific sedation is useful. Either an antipsychotic or a benzodiazepine can be used (Walker 1983).

SIGNS AND SYMPTOMS OF DRUG OVERDOSE IN A PSYCHIATRY SETTING

The emergency psychiatrist should be aware of the possible side-effects of the drugs commonly prescribed in psychiatry. Studies (Baca-García *et al.* 2002) show that among the psychiatric drugs prescribed, benzodiazepines are the drugs used most often for self-poisoning (65% of overdoses), followed by newer antidepressants (11%), tricyclic antidepressants (TCAs) (10%), and antipsychotics (8%).

Benzodiazepine Overdose

An overdose of benzodiazepines affects consciousness and causes disturbances ranging from somnolence to coma. Paradoxical agitation or excitement can occur in some cases. An overdose of benzodiazepines also affects the person's coordination, memory, and cognitive functioning. Benzodiazepines are rarely lethal by themselves, unless respiratory depressants, especially alcohol, barbiturates, and opioids, cause synergism. The management of the patient consists of supportive measures, mainly to maintain the airway, breathing, and circulation. Flumazenil, a benzodiazepine antidote given intravenously in doses not exceeding 1 mg, quickly reverses the effects of benzodiazepines (Alkhouri *et al.* 2010).

Antipsychotic Overdose

Overdoses of typical as well as atypical antipsychotics are seldom fatal unless other drugs are involved. One common effect of an overdose of antipsychotics is depression of the central nervous system. No specific antidote is known to exist, and the management of the patient is mostly supportive. Intravenous crystalloid solutions and peripheral alpha-1-receptor agonists such as phenylephrine and norepinephrine may be used to treat hypotension and reflex tachycardia (Reilly and Kirk 2007).

Antidepressant Overdose

An overdose of tricyclic antidepressants has cardiovascular effects, such as cardiac conduction abnormalities (sinus tachycardia, arrhythmias, and asystole), vasodilatation, and hypotension. Dry mouth, blurred vision, dilated pupils, hyperthermia, and delayed gastric emptying can be attributed to anticholinergic effects. The effects of an overdose of tricyclic antidepressants on the central nervous system are drowsiness, coma, respiratory depression, seizures, and delirium. The assessment of the patient consists of examining serial ECG recordings for the presence of QRS prolongation and QTc prolongation, and a blood gas analysis. The first priority is airway management, with intubation if necessary. This is followed by decontamination using activated charcoal. Even gastric lavage can be considered in the case of potentially life-threatening overdoses, if the patient has arrived within one hour of ingesting the drug. Intravenous fluids should be used to treat hypotension. Seizures should be treated with benzodiazepines, and phenytoin should be avoided (Body *et al.* 2009).

The signs and symptoms of an overdose of the newer antidepressants, especially selective serotonin reuptake inhibitors (SSRIs) which have replaced traditional cyclic antidepressants, are altered mentation or sedation, blurred vision, tremor, nausea, vomiting, hypotension, and tachycardia. Most of these are related to excessive serotonergic stimulation. Rarely, seizures, cardiac conduction disturbances, priapism, and the syndrome of inappropriate antidiuretic hormone secretion (SIADH) occur in addition. Overdoses of the newer antidepressants have also been reported to result in death, though rarely. The management of the patient usually consists of supportive care in which intravenous fluids are used for hypotension and benzodiazepines for agitation. Benzodiazepines and barbiturates constitute the first line of therapy for treating seizures (Reilly and Kirk 2007). The treatment of cardiac conduction disturbances is similar to that in an overdose of tricyclic antidepressants.

Serotonin Syndrome

Excessive stimulation of serotonin (5-HT1A and 5-HT2A) can result in the development of the serotonin syndrome. Altered mental status, autonomic instability, and abnormal neuromuscular activity form the classical triad characterizing the serotonin syndrome. Clonus, agitation, diaphoresis, tremors, and hyperreflexia are the other essential features of the syndrome. The treatment is usually supportive. The offending agent is discontinued, while attempts are made to manage the hyperthermia, muscular rigidity, and agitation. Cooling measures are used to control the hyperthermia, and rigidity and agitation are treated with benzodiazepines. It has been proposed that certain 5-HT2 blockers, such as cyproheptadine, risperidone, and chlorpromazine, be used for the treatment of the serotonin syndrome, but there is not enough valid research to support their use (Reilly and Kirk 2007).

Are Antidepressants Pro-suicide Agents?

In the late 1960s, case reports linked imipramine with worsening of irritability or aggression (Tec and Bindelglas 1968), and other tricyclics were reported to be associated with suicidal ideation (Rampling 1978; Damluji and Ferguson 1998). Observations by Teicher and colleagues (1990) and subsequent case reports by others raised similar concerns in the context of fluoxetine (Dasgupta 1990; Masand, Gupta and Dewan 1991; Wirshing *et al.* 1992). However, a review of the literature by Kapur and colleagues found similar case reports of suicidal behavior among patients taking antipsychotic and anxiolytic medications, and the authors suggested that the very presence of a psychiatric disorder carries a risk of suicidality (Kapur, Mieczkowski and Mann 1992). Two toxicology studies by Isacsson and colleagues (Isacsson *et al.* 1997; Isacsson, Holmgren and Ahlner 2005) also did not support the idea that SSRIs trigger suicide among adults or the youth. Moreover, after three decades of an increase in the overall suicide rate, there has been a reduction in the suicide rate among the youth, averaging about 33% (McCain 2009). Some scientists have attributed this decline to the extensive use of antidepressants (Mann *et al.* 2006). From these pieces of evidence, we conclude that the suicide prevention effects of antidepressants outweigh their pro-suicide effects.

Lithium Overdose

Patients with an acute overdose of lithium may remain asymptomatic despite having much higher levels than the therapeutic levels (0.6–1.2 mEq/L) early after ingestion of the drug. The manifestations of overt lithium overdose include lethargy, confusion, and tremors. Lithium causes T-wave flattening and prolongation of the QT interval. Coma and convulsions may occur at extremely high doses. Permanent neurological impairment may occur in a few patients. However, in most cases the symptoms resolve within a few days to weeks. Nephrogenic diabetes insipidus, neuroleptic malignant syndrome, and serotonin syndrome are the other toxic effects. Lithium must be discontinued, and the treatment consists mainly of fluid therapy and gut decontamination. Gastric lavage and whole bowel irrigation can be considered, the latter especially when the patient has taken an overdose of a sustained-release formulation of lithium. There is only limited evidence supporting the administration of sodium polystyrene sulfonate, which reduces the absorption of lithium and enhances its elimination. This treatment requires additional potassium replacement. Volume restoration is achieved with intravenous administration 1–2 L of normal saline, which is continued at a rate that produces a urine

BOX 6.1 KEY POINTS

- A psychiatric emergency is a defined entity, the emphasis being on the acuteness and severity of behavioral, mood, and thought disturbances that the patient is unable to cope with.
- Accidental overuse, intentional/deliberate misuse, and iatrogenic errors can all result in a drug overdose.
- A drug overdose is the only psychiatric emergency that requires maintaining the airway, breathing, and circulation, all of which need strict medical supervision.
- The commonest psychiatric symptoms resulting from overdoses of the various drugs are altered mental status, seizures, agitation, and psychosis. Violence is another important symptom.
- Among the prescribed psychiatric drugs, benzodiazepines are the drugs used most often for self-poisoning. These are followed by the newer antidepressants, tricyclic antidepressants, and antipsychotics.
- Intentional overdoses are a common cause of completed suicide, and psychotropic drugs are the second most frequently taken drugs that people overdose on to commit suicide. Hence, an emergency psychiatrist must be well versed in suicide assessment and management.
- The suicide prevention effects of antidepressants outweigh their pro-suicide effects.

output of 100 mL/hour (Timmer and Sands 1999). The indications for hemodialysis are a lithium level of >6 mEq/L in any patient, a lithium level of >4 mEq/L in any patient on long-term lithium therapy and a lithium level of 2.5–4.0 mEq/L in any patient with severe neurological symptoms, renal insufficiency, hemodynamic instability or neurological instability (Schwartz and Weathers 2010).

SIDE-EFFECTS OF PSYCHIATRIC DRUGS

In this section, we discuss some of the reactions to drugs used in clinical psychiatry practice. These reactions do not qualify as effects of drug overdose, but require mention as they can cause true emergency situations.

Acute Dystonia

Acute dystonic reactions merit consideration as they are the most common reason for discontinuation of antipsychotics and rare dystonias involving the larynx and esophagus, which are life-threatening. The possibility of laryngeal dystonia should be considered when a patient on antipsychotic therapy presents with acute respiratory distress and stridor. Advanced airway management and even a cricothyroidotomy may be required. The patient should be given supplemental humidified oxygen, along with intravenous centrally acting anticholinergic agents such as diphenhydramine and benztropine. Additionally, benzodiazepines, such as lorazepam, can be given to alleviate anxiety (Reilly and Kirk 2007).

Neuroleptic Malignant syndrome

Neuroleptic malignant syndrome, an idiosyncratic reaction to antipsychotics, is associated with a mortality rate of 4%–30%. It is characterized by hyperthermia, muscle rigidity, autonomic dysfunction, and an altered level of consciousness. Though commonly associated with haloperidol and fluphenazine, the syndrome has been found to occur with all atypical antipsychotics. The laboratory findings in the case of patients with the syndrome are total leukocyte counts ranging from 10,000/mg/L to 40,000/mg/L and elevated serum creatine kinase levels. As neuroleptic malignant syndrome is a life-threatening condition, it is mandatory to abandon the antipsychotic immediately and to initiate aggressive critical care management. Critical care management involves the maintenance of hydration, rapid cooling measures, anticoagulation with low-dose heparin, and advanced airway management. The specific agents used in the treatment of neuroleptic malignant syndrome are dantrolene and bromocriptine (Reilly and Kirk 2007).

Akathisia

Among the psychotropic drugs, it is antipsychotics that most often cause akathisia, though SSRIs can also do so. Akathisia necessarily has two aspects: (i) a subjective report of restlessness or inner tension, applicable particularly to the legs and (ii) objective manifestations of restlessness in the form of semi-purposeful or purposeless movements of the limbs, shifting body position or moving while standing. The risk of akathisia increases with the dose of the antipsychotic or SSRI. The high incidence of akathisia, the marked distress associated with it, and the increased risk of violence and suicide make it a significant psychiatric emergency. Atypical antipsychotics are less likely to cause akathisia. The treatment consists of modifying the antipsychotic regimen. Beta-blockers, such as propranolol, are the most established form of treatment, while benzodiazepines, too, are helpful (Chopra and Smith 1974).

SIGNS AND SYMPTOMS OF SUBSTANCE OVERDOSE

This subject is discussed in Chapter 2.

DRUG OVERDOSE AND SUICIDE

This subject is covered in Chapter 8.

REFERENCES

Alao, AO and Yolles, JC 1998, Isoniazid-induced psychosis. *Ann Pharmacother,* 9, 889–891.

Alkhouri, I, Gibbons, P, Ravindranath, R, *et al.* 2010, Substance-related psychiatric emergencies. In: Riba, M.B., Ravindranath, D. (eds). *Clinical manual of emergency psychiatry*, pp. 187–206. Washington DC: American Psychiatric Publishing, Inc.

Antai-Otong, D 2001, *Psychiatric emergencies: How to accurately assess and manage the patient in crisis*. Wisconsin: Pesi Healthcare.

Baca-García, E, Diaz-Sastre, C, Saiz-Ruiz, J and de Leon, J 2002, How safe are psychiatric medications after a voluntary overdose? *Eur Psychiatry,* 17, 466–470.

Bhatia, MS and Malik, SC 1995, Psychiatric complications of chloroquine. *Indian Pediatr,* 32, 351–353.

Body, R, Bartram, T, Azam, F, *et al.* 2009, Guideline for the management of tricyclic antidepressant overdose. *Gem Net.* Available at www.secure.collemergencymed.ac.uk

Brown, ES, Khan, DA and Nejtek, VA 1999, Psychiatric side-effects of corticosteroids. *Ann Allergy Asthma Immunol,* 83, 495–504.

Chan, TYK 1999, Pyridoxine ineffective in isoniazid-induced psychosis. *Ann Pharmacother,* 33, 1123–1124.

Chopra, G, Smith, J 1974, Psychotic reactions following cannabis use in east Indians. *Arch Gen Psychiatry,* 30, 24–34.

Damluji, NF and Ferguson, JM 1998, Paradoxical worsening of depressive symptomatology caused by antidepressants. *J Clin Psychopharmacol,* 6, 77–92.

Dasgupta, K 1990, Additional cases of suicidal ideation associated with fluoxetine [Letter]. *Am J Psychiatry,* 147, 1570.

Evans, RL, Khalid, S and Kinney, JL 1984, Antimalarial psychosis revisited. *Arch Dermatol,* 120, 765–767.

Hall, RCW, Popkin, MK and Kirkpatrick, B 1978, Tricyclic exacerbation of steroid psychosis. *J Nerv Ment Dis,* 166, 738–742.

Hall, RC, Popkin, MK, Stickney, SK and Gardner, ER 1979, Presentation of the steroid psychosis. *J Nerv Ment Dis,* 167, 229–236.

Haq, MZ, Mishra, BR, Goyal, N and Sinha, VK 2009, Alpha/beta-Arteether-induced mania in a predisposed adolescent. *Gen Hosp Psychiatry,* 31, 391–393.

Isacsson, G, Holmgren, P, Druid, H and Bergman, U 1997, The utilization of antidepressants a key issue in the prevention of suicide: An analysis of 5281 suicides in Sweden during the period 1992–1994. *Acta Psychiatr Scand,* 96, 94–100.

Isacsson, G, Holmgren, P and Ahlner, J 2005, Selective serotonin reuptake inhibitor antidepressants and the risk of suicide: A controlled forensic database study of 14857 suicides. *Acta Psychiatr Scand,* 111, 286–290.

Jena, S 1999, Psychiatric emergencies. In: Vyas, J.N., Ahuja, N (eds). *Textbook of postgraduate psychiatry*, pp. 521–525. New Delhi: Jaypee.

Jerram, T and Greenhalgh, N 1988, Quinine psychosis. *Br J Psychiatry,* 152, 864.

Kapur, S, Mieczkowski, T and Mann, JJ 1992, Antidepressant medications and the relative risk of suicide attempt and suicide. *J Am Med Assoc,* 268, 3441–3445.

Kukoyi, O and Carney, CP 2003, Curses, madness, and mefloquine. *Psychosomatics,* 44, 339–341.

Lawrence Flick Memorial Tuberculosis Clinic, Philadelphia Tuberculosis Control Program 1998, Guidelines for the management of adverse drug effects of antimycobacterial agents, pp. 26–27.

Lewis, DA and Smith, RE 1983, Steroid-induced psychiatric syndromes: A report of 14 cases and a review of the literature. *J Affect Disord,* 5, 319–332.

Ling, MHM, Perry, PJ and Tsuang, MT 1981, Side-effects of corticosteroid therapy. *Arch Gen Psychiatry,* 38, 471–477.

Mann, JJ, Emslie, G, Baldessarini, RJ, Beardslee, W, Fawcett, JA, Goodwin, FK, Leon, AC, Meltzer, HY, Ryan, ND, Shaffer, D and Wagner, KD 2006, ACNP task force report on SSRIs and suicidal behavior in youth. *Neuropsychopharmacology,* 31, 473–492.

Masand, P, Gupta, S and Dewan, M 1991, Suicidal ideation related to fluoxetine treatment [Letter]. *N Engl J Med,* 324, 420.

McCain, JA 2009, Antidepressants and suicide in adolescents and adults: A public health experiment with unintended consequences? *Pharm Therapeutics,* 34, 355–378.

Meier, CR, Wilcock, K, Jick, SS 2004, The risk of severe depression, psychosis or panic attacks with prophylactic antimalarials. *Drug Saf,* 27, 203–213.

Norra, C, Skobel, E, Breuer, C, Haase, G, Hanrath, P and Hoff, P 2003, Ciprofloxacin-induced acute psychosis in a patient with multidrug-resistant tuberculosis. *Eur Psychiatry,* 18, 262–263.

Olson, KR 2004, Emergency evaluation and treatment. In: Olson, KR (ed). *Poisoning and drug overdose.* 4th ed. pp. 19–25. New York: Lange Medical Books/McGraw–Hill.

Potasman, I, Berry, A and Seligmann, H 2000, Neuropsychiatric problems in 2,500 long-term young travelers to the tropics. *J Travel Med,* 7, 5–9.

Prasad, R, Garg, R and Verma, SK 2998, Isoniazid- and ethambutol-induced psychosis. *Ann Thorac Med,* 3, 149–151.

Rampling, D 1978, Aggression: A paradoxical response to tricyclic antidepressants. *Am J Psychiatry,* 135, 117–118.

Reilly, TH, Kirk, MA 2007, Atypical antipsychotics and newer antidepressants. *Emerg Med Clin N Am,* 25, 477–497.

Salafia, A 1992, Candida. Rifampicin-induced flu syndrome and toxic psychosis. *Indian J Lepr,* 64, 537–539.

Schwartz, P and Weathers, M 2010, The psychotic patient. In: Riba, MB, Ravindranath, D (eds). *Clinical manual of emergency psychiatry*, pp. 115–40. Washington DC: American Psychiatric Publishing.

Siegal, FP 1978, Lithium for steroid-induced psychosis. *N Engl J Med,* 299, 155–156.

Sievers, ML and Herrier, RN 1975, Treatment of acute isoniazid toxicity. *Am J Hosp Pharm,* 32, 202–206.

Snider, DE 1980, Pyridoxine supplementation during isoniazid therapy. *Tubercle,* 61, 191–196.

Tec, L and Bindelglas, PM 1968, The treatment of enuresis with imipramine. *Am J Psychiatry,* 125, 266–267.

Teicher, MH, Glod, C and Cole, JO 1990, Emergence of intense suicidal preoccupation during fluoxetine treatment. *Am J Psychiatry,* 147, 207–210.

Timmer, RT and Sands, JM 1999, Lithium intoxication. *J Am Soc Nephrol,* 10, 666.

Vacheron-Trystram, MN, Braitman, A, Cheref, S and Auffray, L 2004, Antipsychotics in bipolar disorders. *Encephale,* 30, 417–424.

Verghese, C 1988, Quinine psychosis. *Br J Psychiatry,* 153, 575–576.

Walker, JI 1983, Basic concepts of emergency care. In: *Psychiatric emergencies intervention and resolution*, pp. 1–20. London: J.B. Lippincott.

Ward, WQ, Walter-Ryan, WG and Shehi, GM 1985, Toxic psychosis: A complication of antimalarial therapy. *J Am Acad Dermatol,* 12, 863–865.

Weinke, T, Trautmann, M, Held, T, Weber, G, Eichenlaub, D, Fleischer, K, Kern, W and Pohle, HD 1991, Neuropsychiatric side-effects after the use of mefloquine. *Am J Trop Med Hyg,* 45, 86–91.

Wirshing, WC, Van Putten, T, Rosenberg, J, Marder, S, Ames, D and Hicks-Gray, T 1992, Fluoxetine, akathisia and suicidality: Is there a causal connection? *Arch Gen Psychiatry,* 49, 580–591.

7 Psychiatric Emergencies in Women

Juliet E.M. Nakku

INTRODUCTION

The several stages of reproductive and hormonal cycles that women go through make them more vulnerable than men to psychological stress and, therefore, to psychiatric emergencies as well. Women find themselves in mental health emergency situations especially during pregnancy and childbirth, in which there is an interplay between a host of conditions. Such situations put both the mother and her newborn baby at risk of ill health, injury, or death. In order to avert the risks, it is imperative for health professionals to be aware of such emergency situations in women. This chapter deals largely with such situations in women.

SEVERE MENTAL ILLNESS IN PREGNANCY

The annual incidence of a psychiatric event during pregnancy is thought to be much lower than that during the non-pregnant period. Hormonal changes during pregnancy may be responsible for modifying the susceptibility to psychiatric events in pregnancy. Mild to moderate forms of common mental disorders occur in 7%–12% of pregnant women (Bennet *et al.* 2004).

Severe psychiatric illness can occur for the first time during pregnancy, but the episode is more commonly a recurrence of a pre-existing mental disorder, such as bipolar affective disorder (mania or depression) or schizophrenia. When this occurs, it increases the risk of a poor perinatal outcome, and hence must be treated as an emergency. Studies of women who suffer from schizophrenia and who develop episodes of psychosis during pregnancy indicate that they have a high risk of giving birth to babies with a low birth-weight (OR 4.3, 95% CI 2.9–6.6) and of stillbirth (OR 4.4, 95% CI 1.4–13.8), even after controlling for smoking and other maternal factors, such as age, parity, education, and pregnancy-induced hypertension (Nilsson *et al.* 2002). The other risks include preterm delivery, the baby being too small for the gestational age and relatively low Apgar scores.

The poor outcome may be mediated by the following risk factors:

- delayed recognition of pregnancy
- less prenatal care
- failure to recognize labor

- a greater incidence of obstetric complications
- psychotic denial of pregnancy, a condition in which the woman denies that she is pregnant despite clear indications, and thus refuses prenatal care, misinterprets signs of labor, risks precipitous and unassisted delivery, and fails to bond with the baby
- smoking, the prevalence of which is high among women with schizophrenia, and
- fewer antenatal care visits.

MANAGEMENT

- A thorough assessment of the mental and physical health of the woman needs to be made (*see* Chapter 3).
- Medication forms a part of the optimal treatment plan as the risk posed to the mother and fetus by not treating the mother almost always outweighs the benefit of withholding medication.
- Imparting psychoeducation to the woman and her partner may minimize the delusional misinterpretation of the changes occurring during pregnancy and help the mother recognize signs of complications of pregnancy and labor.

TREATMENT GUIDELINES

In planning the treatment, one needs to be aware of certain pharmacotherapeutic considerations relevant to the pregnant woman and fetus.

The woman

There is an alteration of pharmacokinetics across the three trimesters of pregnancy.

- The volume of plasma increases by about 50% during pregnancy and body fat also increases, expanding the volume of drug distribution.
- The blood flow to the kidneys rises, as does the glomerular filtration rate, which speeds up renal elimination.
- Many liver enzymes are activated during pregnancy, so drugs are metabolized more quickly, which increases the rate of clearance.

Ultimately, drug concentration is lowered during pregnancy.

The Fetus

- Virtually all psychotropic drugs pass through the placenta.
- Fetal circulation, compared with maternal circulation, contains less protein. This leaves more of the drug unbound, which facilitates entry into the fetal brain.
- Liver enzymes are relatively inactive in the fetus, increasing the possibility of toxic effects.
- Excretion is relatively prolonged.
- The blood–brain barrier is incomplete and the nervous system immature, and, therefore, more sensitive to the effects of drugs.

The above predispose the fetus to the risk of teratogenesis, which needs to be avoided as far as possible. In addition, it is necessary to minimize interference with the smooth progress of labor and delivery, prevent withdrawal effects in the neonate, and avoid effects on the infant's neurodevelopment in the future. There are inconclusive reports of the occurrence of all the above. As such, the following guidelines should be kept in mind.

- As far as possible, one should consider monotherapy with the lowest effective dose of the drug, taking care not to undertreat the woman, as this increases the risk of exposure for the fetus without giving the mother the benefit of recovery.
- Medication should be given for the shortest period necessary.
- Drugs known to have adverse effects on the fetus should be avoided as far as possible. In the first trimester, exposure to low-potency phenothiazines, lithium carbonate, and anticonvulsants should be avoided as these have been found to be teratogenic (Brockington *et al.* 2011). Benzodiazepines should be avoided when labor is imminent as they may interfere with the progress of labor. These drugs are not absolutely contraindicated in pregnancy. Lithium carbonate may be initiated or restarted after the first trimester if it is deemed the best choice. It may also replace anticonvulsants as a mood stabilizer.
- The pregnant woman and her family must be counseled on the treatment options so that they can make an informed choice.

DEPRESSION WITH SUICIDE

The prevalence of depression among pregnant women is approximately 10%. Women who may be at greater risk for depression during pregnancy include those who are young, are ambivalent about the pregnancy, have a personal or family history of depression, and are experiencing marital problems. The symptoms of depression during pregnancy are consistent with those found at other times in a woman's life. However, it is often difficult for clinicians and patients to distinguish the cause of neurovegetative symptoms, such as fatigue, disruption of sleep, weight gain, changes in appetite, loss of energy, and decreased concentration. Each of these hallmark symptoms of depression, in isolation, can be a simple effect of pregnancy. Therefore, many women disregard their depressive symptoms, believing them to be a normal part of pregnancy. To ensure that there is neither underdiagnosis nor overdiagnosis of depression, the number and severity of the symptoms, as well as their relationship to stressors and mood and physical changes, must be thoroughly assessed. A thorough assessment of the risk factors, the woman's feelings about the pregnancy, her future plans, her mood, and her level of anxiety is critical for distinguishing the cause of the neurovegetative symptoms. Although pregnancy appears to be a time when the risk of suicide is lower than usual, the risk of self-harm, suicide attempts, and completed suicide does exist in the case of some women. Thus, suicidality must be assessed in any depressed woman, regardless of their pregnancy status.

SUICIDE IN THE PERINATAL PERIOD

Pregnant women may at times become suicidal,which poses a challenge in their

BOX 7.1 RISK FACTORS OF SUICIDE IN PREGNANT WOMEN

- The nature of psychiatric symptoms including depression, anxiety, and psychosis
- A feeling of hopelessness and helplessness
- A history of substance use or abuse
- A previous history of suicide
- The individual's personality traits and tendency to impulsivity
- Current and past psychosocial stressors
- Comorbid physical illness
- Family history of suicide

BOX 7.2 ASSESSMENT OF SUICIDAL INTENT

- A strong wish to die
- Ready availability of lethal means to die, e.g. gun, rope
- Ambivalence
- Frequency and intensity of thoughts of death
- Repeated warnings about dying or killing oneself
- A suicide note

management. The risk of suicide in pregnant depressed women is up to 5% (Lindahl, Pearson and Colpe 2005). Therefore, it is important to always assess risk of suicide in such women with mental health problems. The assessment of risk of suicide starts with a full psychiatric evaluation of the woman (Box 7.1) (Jacobs 2007). Further evaluation of suicide should include an assessment of suicide intent or imminent suicide (Box 7.2). (Suicide risk assessment has been discussed in detail in Chapter 8.)

The management of suicide in pregnant women is complex. Recommended drugs to reduce suicide risk include benzodiazepines in case of severe anxiety, antipsychotics in case of psychosis, antidepressants in case of depression, and lithium carbonate in case of bipolar disorder. There is little or no evidence to support the safety of these treatments in pregnant and postpartum women. However, electroconvulsive therapy has been shown to be efficacious in reducing acute suicidal behavior and to be safe. Its long-term benefit has not been established.

BIPOLAR DISORDER WITH AGITATION AND AGGRESSION IN PREGNANCY

Bipolar I disorder affects 1%–2% of the population and is equally distributed among men and women. Women with bipolar disorder tend to experience a greater number of depressed, mixed, and rapid-cycling episodes than men. Many women with bipolar disorder experience an episode during their childbearing years and appear to be at the greatest risk during the perinatal period. Retrospective studies originally suggested that the risk of recurrence of a mood episode is lower among women with bipolar disorder. However, this is controversial.

Recent studies have found that the rates of relapse during pregnancy were high among women who had bipolar disorder and discontinued their medication. The rates of the occurrence of a recurrent affective episode were similar for pregnant and non-pregnant women who discontinued maintenance lithium. Except for a history of chronic depression and the discontinuation of medications (especially rapid discontinuation), the risk factors for an episode of depression or mania during pregnancy among women with bipolar disorder have not yet been established.

Because of the high risk of teratogenicity associated with many mood stabilizers, women may abruptly discontinue their medications or be advised to do so during or in preparation for pregnancy. The dose of some medications may actually need to be increased during pregnancy to maintain stability of mood. Affective symptoms may recur because of inadequate treatment, since health providers and mothers often try to minimize fetal exposure to the medication. Emergency physicians often come across women presenting with depression, mania, or a mixed episode of abrupt onset owing to such medication-related issues. Decisions regarding whether to increase or restart medications are complicated, and a comprehensive risk–benefit analysis is of critical importance. Generally for a pregnant woman with untreated mania, the risk of a poor obstetric outcome is great. It is recommended to start or restart treatment immediately. An antipsychotic such as haloperidol or olanzapine is preferable. However, after the first trimester, mood stabilizers such as lithium carbonate or sodium valproate may be restarted if these previously kept the woman well.

The management of aggression and agitation in pregnancy is a complex undertaking. While the management of acutely disturbed patients has been described, there is very little literature to guide the management of such patients if they are pregnant or postpartum. Both medication (rapid tranquilization) and physical restraining may be used. However, these can pose serious risks to the safety of the woman and the growing fetus. The aggression or agitation episode often causes distress, which may precipitate the excessive secretion of adrenalin and cortisol that may result in cardiac rhythm disturbances. Worse still, few or no studies have been done to guide on the safety profile of such treatment in pregnancy

Medication for Aggressive Agitated Pregnant Women

To the extent possible, negotiation and techniques to calm the patient down should be used. These may not work at times, requiring the use of medication; in such cases rapid tranquilization may be the option. The following preliminary measures should be taken whenever possible (Kirkley 2014):

- Monitor the woman's temperature, blood pressure, pulse, and respiration
- Do a pretreatment ECG.

When choosing an agent for rapid tranquilization consider an antipsychotic or benzodiazepine with a shorter half-life (e.g. haloperidol or lorazepam).

- The minimum effective dose should be given to minimize the risk of neonatal adverse effects, e.g. neonatal extrapyramidal symptoms in case of an antipsychotic or floppy baby syndrome in case of a benzodiazepine.

- Haldol (5–10 mg) and/or lorazepam (1–2 mg) singly or in combination are by far the most commonly used and recommended in pregnancy and the postpartum woman.
- Repeat same dose every 30–45 minutes if the woman does not calm down up to a total of three doses
- The woman should be managed in close collaboration with a pediatrician and anesthetist.
- Other drugs that may be used include olanzapine, risperidone, and diazepam.

Restraint of Aggressive Agitated Pregnant Women

Restraint must be used only as a last option in aggressive and agitated women. The safety and rights of the woman and fetus must be borne in mind: The following guidelines must be considered (NSW Government 2012):

- Holding a pregnant patient in the seated position is safer than in any other position.
- If there is need to lie them down, pregnant patients should be positioned in the left lateral position (on her left side) to reduce the likelihood of compression of the aorta and vena cava.
- Do not restrain the pregnant woman in the supine position for extended periods of time.
- Avoid restraining in the prone position as this could lead to airway obstruction and respiratory distress.
- Identify and manage any medical risk factors.
- Observe the patient every 15 minutes for the first hour and every 30–45 minutes thereafter till she calms down.

POSTPARTUM PSYCHOSIS

Introduction

Postpartum psychosis, also called puerperal psychosis, is a serious mental condition. It is an acute and florid disturbance of mood, thought, perception, and behavior, occurring among women soon after childbirth. It is rare, occurring in 1–2/1000 live-births (Chaudron and Robertson-Blackmore 2005). Fifty to sixty percent of the sufferers are often first-time mothers (Bhattacharya and Vyas 1969; Brockington 2004). The onset of postpartum psychosis is within days to weeks of delivery. Most episodes start within 2–4 weeks and nearly all will have started within 8 weeks of childbirth. Postpartum psychosis is characterized by mood symptoms, delusions, and thoughts of self-harm or inflicting harm on the baby. While it puts the mother and her infant at risk of harm or death, it may also pose a danger to other people around the sick mother. The fifth edition of the Diagnostic and Statistical Manual of Mental Disorders (DSM-5, American Psychiatric Association 2013) terms postpartum psychosis as bipolar disorders with peripartum onset under the unspecified "Bipolar and related disorders" (code 296.80).

In the United Kingdom, an inquiry into maternal deaths showed that suicide was the leading cause of maternal mortality, accounting for 28% of maternal deaths. The majority of those who died due to suicide suffered from postpartum psychosis. Gibson (1982) estimated that 62% of mothers who commit infanticide go on to commit suicide. Because of these serious consequences, early diagnosis and management of postpartum psychosis is imperative.

Causes

The cause of puerperal psychosis is not known, but biological, including genetic, and hormonal factors may play a role. This is thought to be more true of postpartum psychosis than postpartum depression because the onset of psychosis is closer to childbirth than that of depression. The episodes of psychosis may be triggered by both organic and non-organic factors. The most significant risk factor is having had a previous episode of psychosis. Other risk factors are listed in Box 7.3.

Evaluation

The evaluation of a patient who appears to present with postpartum psychosis is aimed at identifying the predominant symptoms and the factors associated with them. The evaluation entails the following:

- It must be established that the woman has had a baby in the last 6–8 weeks.
- It is necessary to find out about the onset of the symptoms. The onset of postpartum psychosis is often within the first 4 weeks of the delivery, but the mother may present to medical services much later. The symptoms start acutely and are usually florid.
- A brief assessment must be made to establish the predominant psychiatric symptoms/problems. Information may be obtained from a relative as well as from the woman herself (Box 7.4).
- A general physical examination must always be conducted to check for any physical manifestations which may accompany the psychosis or which may even indicate a possible physical cause. One should, for example, look out for fever, dehydration, dyspnea, anemia, possible points of infection, and high blood pressure.
- The wellness of the baby, if present, should be assessed.
- If possible, a full psychiatric assessment should be made or the patient should be referred to psychiatric services for a detailed assessment.

BOX 7.3 RISK FACTORS FOR POSTPARTUM PSYCHOSIS

- Previous personal history of psychosis
- Family history of psychosis
- Previous history of postpartum psychosis
- Primiparity
- Young age
- Poor social support
- Physical ill health
- Substance abuse

BOX 7.4 USUAL PSYCHIATRIC SYMPTOMS

- Extreme agitation
- Sleep disturbances
- Appetite disturbances
- Confusion which may be rapidly changing
- Depressed mood or periods of euphoria
- Lability of mood
- Delusions, usually centering around the baby
- Auditory or visual hallucinations
- Indecisiveness, especially with regard to caring for the baby
- Thoughts of suicide or infanticide

Many researchers (Brockington 1996; Kendell, Chalmers and Platz 1987) have found that manic symptoms predominate in most patients with postpartum psychosis. Some patients, however, present with depression with psychotic features, schizophreniform features or organic features. Quite frequently, the picture is mixed – the patient has symptoms that suggest all the above syndromes to some degree and the symptoms change rapidly, from hour to hour (Gibson 1982). The delusions often relate to the baby, but may be paranoid.

Differential Diagnosis

Many conditions may give rise to symptoms that simulate postpartum psychosis or may underlie postpartum psychosis symptomatology. These include psychotic disorder due to a general medical condition. While many women suffer non-organic postpartum mental illness, it is important to be mindful of and to rule out organic causes of psychosis in the postpartum period. Infection is one such cause. Bhattacharya and Vyas (1969) found that 76% of a sample of 50 women with postpartum psychosis had an infection and they suggested a predominant puerperal sepsis etiology at the time. We must note, however, that with the many advances in medicine and the advent of antibiotics, infectious causes are no longer as common, but they are nevertheless a possibility. In developing countries where the rate of HIV/AIDs infection is high, secondary mania or depression may occur postpartum in infected women.

Patil *et al.* (2010) describe a 30-year-old woman with psychosis and primary hypoparathyroidism. Her parathyroid hormone levels did not improve on correction of her serum magnesium. Her psychosis improved when the serum calcium was corrected. The other conditions that have been cited to be associated with the onset of postpartum psychosis as listed in Box 7.5 (Chaudron and Robertson-Blackmore 2005; Brockington 2004).

Management

The goals of management are: Crisis resolution and to find dispositional solutions (i.e. what should be done with the woman after the crisis resolves, i.e. the individualized

BOX 7.5 DIFFERENTIAL DIAGNOSIS OF POSTPARTUM PSYCHOSIS

- Infection
- Substance withdrawal
- Hormonal disorders
- Toxemia
- Neoplasm
- Cerebral venous thrombosis
- Chorea gravidarum
- Heart disease
- Postpartum recurrence of major psychiatric disorder in previously affected individuals

after care needed after the period of crises, e.g. living arrangement, child care, longer term hospitalization and treatment, etc.)

Treatment

- *Hospital admission:* As far as possible, postpartum psychosis should be treated in hospital. The mother runs the risk of harming or neglecting herself and poses a danger to her infant, and often, her other children and family members. Dobson and Sales (2000) report that acutely psychotic women are responsible for 25% of all infanticide cases in which the infant has crossed 24 hours of life. Postpartum psychosis often constitutes a crisis for the family. Removing the patient from her home and admitting her to hospital may be the first step in resolving the crisis. Further, the symptoms evolve and change so rapidly, and sometimes unpredictably, that constant observation is necessary over a period of time.

If the first encounter with the patient is in an emergency ward, she should be transferred to a mental health unit where she can be admitted for further care. The mother should be admitted together with her baby if mother–baby services are available or if they can be improvised. This ensures that bonding is not disrupted. However, the mother's interaction with the baby and breastfeeding may initially need to be supervised to prevent harm to the baby, in case the mother develops ideas of harming the baby.

- *Medication:* Antipsychotics, such as haloperidol, are the treatment of choice. A mood stabilizer or antidepressant, such as any selective serotonin reuptake inhibitor (SSRI), may be needed in addition. The former would be needed if the predominant syndrome is mania and the latter if it is depression.

If a woman had episodes of mood disorder which were treated with lithium carbonate prior to pregnancy, the treatment may be reinstated after the first trimester. The baby will, however, need to be monitored closely in the days and weeks immediately after delivery for any signs of lethergy, restlessness, or poor feeding, which may rarely occur as signs of infant lithium toxicity.

- *Social issues:* Adequate attention must be paid to the family of the patient, i.e. her spouse, infant, other children, and close relatives. Postpartum psychosis in the family constitutes a crisis and can be overwhelming. The family members suffer a great deal of anxiety, and there is a lot of uncertainty in terms of what to do and what will happen to the mother and the baby. Efforts should be made to explain what is going on and how to best manage the mother and baby.
- *Physical treatments:* In mothers with severe affective symptoms (mania or depression), electroconvulsive therapy is efficacious (Chaudron and Robertson-Blackmore 2005; Doucet *et al.* 2011) and may hasten recovery. It is also safe.
- *Prevention:* For women who have had previous episodes of or who have received treatment for postpartum psychosis or non-pregnancy-related mood disorders, treatment with antipsychotics or mood stabilizers may be reinstated early in the postpartum period if it had earlier been discontinued during pregnancy.

Prognosis

About 30%–60% of women with postpartum psychosis develop further episodes (Andrews and Jenkins 1999; Moses-Kolko and Feintuch 2002). Most of these occur during the periods when they are not pregnant, while at least 25% are episodes that recur during pregnancy (Scottish Intercollegiate Guideline Network 2002).

Postpartum Anxiety Disorders

Anxiety disorders have not usually been considered as among the postpartum disorders. However, in the clinical situation, comorbid anxiety disorders or severe anxiety symptoms often go hand in hand with mood disorders. In addition, the obsessive thinking and compulsive behaviors often displayed by women in the postpartum period mandate clinicians to consider anxiety disorders, including obsessive–compulsive disorder (OCD), generalized anxiety disorder, and panic disorder.

Women may experience either an anxiety disorder of new onset or an exacerbation of an existing anxiety disorder in the postpartum period. For some women who have OCD or a spectrum of OCD symptoms, the arrival of a new infant who requires the mother to be increasingly flexible can be very distressing. It is important to inquire about habits related to cleaning and orderliness because these can give one a clue about the difficulty some women may experience when a new infant interrupts their rituals or schedules. While there are no studies specifically dealing with the treatment of OCD during the perinatal period, the established approach of cognitive behavioral therapy, as well as the use of an SSRI, is recommended. The use of SSRIs for postpartum anxiety disorders involves the same concerns as those involved in the case of postpartum depression.

Pregnancy Loss

Therapeutic abortions and spontaneous pregnancy losses are often lumped together when the relationship between pregnancy loss and mental health is considered. Each event can affect a woman's mental health. No one event should be assumed to be of lesser or greater magnitude than another. The rate of depression among women who have undergone therapeutic terminations of pregnancy has not been established. While data indicate no increase in serious psychiatric sequelae, the risk of depression after a therapeutic termination is greater among women who have a history of psychiatric illness, feel coerced into the termination, are ambivalent about the termination, and have limited social support.

Miscarriage, defined as an involuntary pregnancy loss before 20 weeks' gestation, is relatively common, occurring in 15%–25% of recognized pregnancies. In contrast, perinatal loss, defined as an involuntary loss after 20 weeks' gestation, is relatively rare, occurring in 1.2% of pregnancies. The relative risk for an episode of major depression within 6 months of a pregnancy loss is 2.5, but it is as high as 5 among women who do not have other living children. Among women with a history of depression, more than half will experience a recurrence of depression in the 6 months after a pregnancy loss. Another risk factor for the development of depression after a pregnancy loss is being relatively older. The gestational age of the fetus at the time of the loss is an additional factor.

Following a pregnancy loss, some women may visit a doctor immediately, grieving severely and in an acute crisis. Others, however, may not see a doctor for weeks or months. Women are often not prepared for the extent of grief that they experience. Women who have had repeated miscarriages may run a greater risk of developing depression because of the repeated roller-coaster of hope and grief. Miscarriages and therapeutic terminations are often considered a private matter that is discussed only among the couple and medical providers, so many women do not receive the kind of support they would have received from family and friends in the case of other deaths or losses.

In contrast, perinatal losses, including stillbirths, are often very public losses because many pregnancies are obvious at the time of the loss. Women suffering perinatal losses may have more support but are often faced with questions about the baby and the delivery from persons who are not close to them. It may be difficult for the woman to repeatedly discuss the loss. Anniversary dates that may precipitate crises include the anniversary of the birth/loss, as well as the anniversary of the original anticipated birth date. The birth of a subsequent child can also be a trigger for bereavement and even depression for some women who are still grieving a previous pregnancy loss. Many women who may require treatment for depression or anxiety after a pregnancy loss wish to become pregnant again as soon as possible. Special consideration is often required when choosing medication for these women.

REFERENCES

Andrews, G and Jenkins, R (eds) 1999, Puerperal psychosis: In: *Management of mental disorders* (UK edition). Sydney: World Health Organization Collaborating Center for Mental Health and Substance Abuse.

Bennet, HA, Einarson, A, Taddio, A, Koren, G and Einarson, TR 2004, Prevalence of depression during pregnancy: Systematic review. *Obstet Gynecol,* 103, 698–709.

Bhattacharya, D and Vyas, JN 1969, Puerperal psychosis. *Indian J Psychiatry,* 11, 38–39.

Brockington, I 1996, *Motherhood and mental health.* Oxford: Oxford University Press.

Brockington, I 2004, Diagnosis and management of post-partum disorders: A review. *World Psychiatry,* 3, 89–95.

Brockington, I, Chandra, P, Dubowitz, H, Jones, D, Moussa, S, Nakku, J and Quadros Ferre, I 2011, WPA guidance on the protection and promotion of mental health in children of persons with severe mental disorders. *World Psychiatry,* 10, 93–102.

Chaudron, HL and Robertson-Blackmore, E 2005, Differential diagnosis of postpartum psychosis. Psychiatric issues in emergency care settings, *Psychiatric Times,* Vol 4, No 4.

Dobson, V and Sales, B 2000, The science of infanticide and mental illness. *Psychology, Public Policy, and Law,* 6, 1098–1112.

Doucet, S, Jones, I, Letourneau, N, Dennis, CL and Blackmore, ER 2011, Interventions for the prevention and treatment of postpartum psychosis: A systematic review. *Arch Womens Ment Health,* 14, 89–98.

DSM-5 American Psychiatric Association 2013, Diagnostic and statistical manual of mental disorders. Arlington: American Psychiatric Publishing.

Gibson, E 1982, *Homicide in England and Wales*, 1967–1971. London: Pitman.

Jacobs, D 2007, Suicide assessment. University of Michigan Depression Center Colloquium Series [PowerPoint presentation]. Available at www.stopasuicide.org/professional.aspx

Kendell, RE, Chalmers, JC and Platz, C 1987, Epidemiology of puerperal psychoses. *Br J Psychiatry,* 150, 662–673.

Kirkley, C 2014, Policy for the Rapid Tranquilisation (RT) of Adult Patients Displaying Acutely Disturbed or Violent Behaviour. Available at http://www.qegateshead.nhs.uk/sites/default/files/users/user10/RM80%20Policy%20for%20Rapid%20Tranquilisation%20v1.pdf

Lindahl, V, Pearson, JL and Colpe, L 2005, Prevalence of suicidality during pregnancy and the postpartum. *Arch Womens Ment Health,* 8, 77–87.

Moses-Kolko, EL and Feintuch, MG 2002, Perinatal psychiatric disorders: A clinical review. *Curr Prob Obst Gyne,* 25, 61–112.

Nilsson, E, Lichtenstein, P, Cnattingius, S, Murray, RM and Hultman, CM 2002, Women with schizophrenia: Pregnancy outcome and infant death among their offspring. *Schizophr Res,* 58, 221–229.

NSW Government, Ministry of Health 2012, Aggression, seclusion, and restraint in mental health facilities in NSW. A policy document. Available at http://www.health.nsw.gov.au/policies/pd/2012/pdf/PD2012_035.pdf

Patil, NJ, Yadav, SS, Gokhale, YA and Padwa, N 2010, Primary hypoparathyroidism: Psychosis in postpartum period. *J Assoc Physicians India,* 58, 506–508.

Scottish Intercollegiate Guideline Network 2002, Postpartum depression and puerperal pychosis. A National Clinical Guideline.

8 Emergency Management of Suicidal Behavior

Lakshmi Vijayakumar,
Vinayak Vijayakumar

INTRODUCTION

Suicide is a global public health problem. Each year, approximately 80,000 individuals die of suicide worldwide, 10–20 million attempt suicide, and 50–120 million are profoundly affected by the suicide or attempted suicide of a close relative or associate. The global suicide rate is estimated to be 11.4/100,000, that for males being 15/100,000 and that for females 8/100,000 (World Suicide Report 2014). Suicide represented 1.8% of the global burden of disease in 1998 and this figure is expected to increase to 2.4% in 2020 (Bertolote and Fleischmann 2009). Suicide is the second leading cause of mortality in young persons in the age group of 15–24 years (accounting for 6.3% of all deaths) and the first leading cause in the case of females between the ages of 15 and 19 years (accounting for 8.2% of all deaths) (Patton *et al.* 2009).

Psychiatric emergencies represent approximately 10% of all emergencies faced by the physician, and constitute the third most frequent cause of emergencies after internal and surgical causes. This is corroborated by a validated questionnaire, in which emergency physicians stated that psychiatric emergencies comprised around 10% of their emergency calls (Pajonk *et al.* 1998). Although data suggest that the prevalence of suicide attempts bringing people to the emergency medical system is low, the clinical relevance is reported to be high when one takes into account the global magnitude of the problem (Pajonk *et al.* 2002).

Shneidman (1985) defines suicide as a conscious act of self-induced annihilation, best understood as a multidimensional malaise in a needful individual who defines an issue for which suicide is perceived as the best solution. According to WHO's definition, suicide is a deliberate act to end one's life.

The four broad categories of suicidality are:

- Suicide
- Attempted suicide
- Suicidal ideation
- Self-harm.

Suicide and suicidal ideation are easily understood, but the terms attempted suicide and self-harm encompass a wide variety of behaviors. The CDC defines a suicide attempt as a non-fatal, self-inflicted potentially injurious behavior, with an intent to die as a result of the behavior. A suicide attempt may or may not result in injury. Non-suicidal self-injurious behavior is a self-inflicted potentially harmful behavior, with the individual having no intent to die as a result of the behavior, such as to affect external circumstances or affect internal state. In many low- and middle-income countries (LAMI), suicide is seen as shameful, sinful, selfish, weak, or manipulative. However, it is condoned in some religious and sociocultural contexts.

EPIDEMIOLOGY

The majority of suicides (76%) in the world occur in LAMI countries (World Suicide Report 2014; Krug *et al.* 2002). In the developed countries, the suicide rate is high in the age group of 15–24 years and the highest among the elderly. The male–female ratio is greater than in LAMI countries, at 3:1 or greater than 3:1. The risk of suicide is relatively higher among the divorced, widowed, and separated. In LAMI countries, the highest rates are often found among the young (below 30 years of age). The male–female ratio is 2:1 (India 1.4:1, China 1:1.3) and married women are at a higher risk. The common methods used in the developed countries are firearms, car exhaust, and poisoning, whereas in LAMI countries, they are pesticide poisoning, hanging, and self-immolation.

RISK AND PROTECTIVE FACTORS

Risk Factors

The risk factors for suicide may be divided into three categories (Rockville 2001):

- *Bio-psychosocial risk factors*, including mental disorders; alcohol or substance use disorders; hopelessness; aggressive tendencies; a history of trauma or abuse; major physical illnesses; a family history of suicide; and previous suicide attempts.
- *Environmental factors including job* and financial losses; relational or social losses; easy access to lethal means; and local clusters of suicide that have a contagious influence.
- *Sociocultural factors*, including lack of social support and sense of isolation; stigma associated with help-seeking behavior; barriers to accessing healthcare, especially treatment for mental health and substance abuse; certain cultural and religious beliefs (for instance, the belief that suicide represents a noble resolution of a personal dilemma); and exposure to, including through the media, and the influence of others who have died by suicide.

Protective Factors

- Effective clinical care for mental, physical, and substance use disorders
- Restricted access to highly lethal means of suicide
- Easy access to a variety of clinical interventions and support for help-seeking
- Strong connections with and support from the family and community

- Support through ongoing medical and mental healthcare relationships
- Skills in problem-solving and conflict resolution, and non-violent handling of disputes
- Cultural and religious beliefs that discourage suicide and support self-preservation.

PRESENTATION OF THE SUICIDAL PATIENT

A potentially suicidal patient can present to the emergency department (ED) in the following ways:

- Overtly suicidal patients who either come on their own or are brought by others in search of help
- Patients who have just attempted suicide
- Those presenting with other psychiatric or substance abuse disorders.

The third category of patients might also include covertly suicidal patients who come to the ED complaining of various problems. Such patients may present with a confusing array of signs and symptoms. Assessing them can be quite challenging and their potential to commit suicide often goes unassessed. They could present with somatic complaints or have an undiagnosed underlying psychiatric disorder, such as depression or panic disorder (Buzan and Weissberg 1992). Thus, when evaluating vague or unexplainable physical complaints, the clinician must ask about depression, panic attacks, and the potential for suicide. Similarly, patients presenting with psychotic symptoms or symptoms of depression, anxiety, panic attacks, or drug withdrawal could also be covertly suicidal and must be asked about such feelings.

INTERVIEWING THE SUICIDAL PATIENT

Most suicidal patients are willing to discuss their thoughts if asked, but it has been shown that only one in six clinicians inquires into the matter. It is a popular myth that asking a patient about suicide will introduce them to the idea when no such idea existed previously. In cases of attempted suicide, the objective of the initial interview is two-fold: (i) to make use of the chance to collect information and (ii) to provide emotional support to the patient and take advantage of the opportunity to establish a bond with them (Bertolote, de Mello-Santos and Botega 2010). The initial interview often does not take place in a favorable setting. Much of the time, it is in the emergency room and the patient is still reserved, drowsy, or under intensive care. In these conditions, the patient might not be very cooperative and might even deny having attempted to take their own life. One should keep the patient's fragile mental state in mind, and efforts should be made to make them feel at ease and slowly establish a rapport (Bryan and Rudd 2006). A hierarchical approach to questioning has been recommended, that is, the intensity of the interview should be gradually stepped up so that the clinician can perhaps reduce the patient's anxiety or agitation and also improve their rapport with the patient (Bryan and Rudd 2006). A desperate patient with a definite plan for suicide is unlikely to share their dilemma with the clinician even if the latter asks all the right questions but asks them in an insensitive or a demeaning manner (Buzan 1992).

A sequence of useful questions is: Do you feel unhappy and helpless? Do you feel desperate? Are you unable to face each day? Do you feel that life is a burden and not worth living? Do you feel like committing suicide? It is important to ask these questions in a secure and supportive environment, for example:

- After a rapport has been established
- When the patient feels comfortable about expressing their emotions
- When the patient is expressing loneliness, helplessness, hopelessness, despair, etc.

In LAMI countries, the EDs are always overcrowded and the clinician may have to see numerous patients in a short span of time. In such a setting, if the patient seems suicidal, they should be gently asked to wait in a quiet room, not left alone, and be assured that the clinician would like to spend more time with them.

Principles in Risk Assessment

The assessment of the risk of suicide in every person is unique, complex, and challenging. It is an ongoing process, is collaborative, and relies on clinical judgment. The assessment must be made taking all threats, warning signs, and risk factors seriously. Asking difficult and sensitive questions is treatment by itself and can help uncover the underlying message. Assessment is made in a cultural context and must be documented.

IMPORTANT AREAS OF ASSESSMENT (TABLE 8.1)

The assessment process must include:

- Conducting a thorough psychiatric examination in which the risk factors and protective factors are identified, and the risk factors which can be modified are distinguished from those which cannot be modified
- Specifically enquiring about suicidal thoughts, plans, and behaviors
- Establishing the level of the risk of suicide: low, moderate, high
- Determining the treatment setting and plan (Bertolote, de Mello-Santos and Botega 2010).

One can obtain a holistic picture of the patient's problems and be better able to determine the risk of their committing suicide, as well as the treatment plan, by assessing the current presentation of suicidality (method, circumstances, and intentionality); epidemiological data (risk factors and relevant events); predisposing and precipitating factors; the individual and family history; and the patient's physical health and social support system. One must also look for the presence of psychiatric illness, and examine individual and personality factors (Bertolote, de Mello-Santos and Botega 2010).

Psychiatric Examination

The psychiatric disorders that are associated with an increased risk of suicide are (i) mood disorders, (ii) alcohol and substance use disorders, (iii) psychotic disorders, (iv) anxiety disorders, and (v) personality disorders (particularly borderline and antisocial

TABLE 8.1

Areas to Evaluate in the Assessment of Suicidal Behaviors

Current presentation of suicidality	• Suicidal or self-harming thoughts, plans, behaviors, and intent
Symptomatic presentation	• Evidence of hopelessness, impulsiveness, anhedonia, panic attacks, or anxiety
Psychiatric illness	• Current signs and symptoms of psychiatric disorders • Look for comorbidities in particular
History	• Past history of suicidal behavior • Past history of psychiatric illness • Past medical history/ surgical history • Family history of suicidal behavior and mental illness, including substance use
Psychosocial situation	• Acute or chronic psychological stressors • Social support systems • Cultural and religious beliefs about suicide
Individual factors	• Personality traits • Coping skills • Past responses to stress

Source: Bryan and Rudd 2006, APA guidelines

personality disorders). Psychiatric disorders are often chronic and hence, it is important to have a knowledge of the symptoms and situations which increase the risk of suicide.

Mood Disorders

Specific symptoms that increase the risk of suicide are hopelessness, severe anxiety and panic, anhedonia, and psychotic symptoms. In LAMI countries, the majority of persons who are suffering from depression and commit suicide take their lives in their very first episode of depression. The clinician should be aware that in LAMI countries, even a young person who is going through his first episode of mild or moderate depression is at risk of suicide.

Alcohol and Substance Use Disorder

Alcohol abuse and dependence is an important risk factor for suicide in many LAMI countries. Suicide often occurs late in the course of the disease as by that time, the habit has taken a heavy toll on the person's health, financial affairs, as well as social, interpersonal, economic, and occupational functioning.

Psychotic Disorders

In schizophrenia, suicide occurs early in the course of the illness, as well as during early recovery and early relapse. Depressive symptoms, a higher level of functioning, insight into the functional deficits caused by the disorder, violent or command hallucinations, agitation, akathasia, and recent discharge from hospital are associated with an increased risk.

According to the American Association of Suicidology consensus reached on the warning signs of suicidal behavior, the signs include (Rudd *et al.* 2006):

- Hopelessness
- Rage, anger, seeking revenge
- Acting reckless or engaging in risky activities, seemingly without thinking
- Feeling trapped, as if there is no way out
- Increasing alcohol or drug abuse
- Withdrawing from friends, family, or society
- Anxiety, agitation, inability to sleep, or sleeping all the time
- Dramatic changes in mood
- Seeing no reason for living, having no sense of purpose in life

Most developing nations tend to view suicide as a social problem. Mental illness, which is seen as one of the causes of suicide, is given an equal conceptual status as love affairs, family conflict, and social maladjustment. In developing countries, suicide is preceded by a period of acute stress. One can almost always identify certain major life events that have occurred in the two weeks preceding a suicide attempt. Chronic stress has also been identified as one of the reasons for suicide. Stress can result from financial setbacks, grief over the death of a loved one, academic failure, the break-up of a marriage, and other environmental and sociocultural factors. Poverty, poor physical health, and physical and psychological abuse, among other factors, increase the risk for suicide.

Assessment of Lethality and Intent (Specific Enquiry Regarding Plan, Method)

Measures of suicidal intent and lethality are commonly used to determine the seriousness of suicide attempts. The level of suicidal intent, defined as the degree to which the individual wished to die at the time of the attempt (Harriss, Hawton and Zahl 2005), is a powerful predictor of completed suicide and can be easily assessed in clinical settings. Lethality is defined as the seriousness of the physical consequences of or the risk posed to life by the suicide attempt. The lethality of the plan can be ascertained through questions about the method, the patient's knowledge and skill concerning its use, and the presence or absence of intervening persons or protective circumstances (Table 8.2) (Jacobs *et al.* 2003).

Establishing the Level of Suicide Risk (Low, Medium, High)

The assessment of the risk of suicide is based on a comprehensive assessment of the risk factors for suicide and the warning signs, as well as an appraisal of the protective factors that could mitigate the risk (Granello 2010). In LAMI countries, clinicians work in an under-resourced environment and are overworked, which makes them tend to overlook subtle signs of suicidal thoughts and behaviors, or to conduct only a cursory assessment. A thorough assessment can be made in 20–40 minutes (Table 8.3).

TABLE 8.2

Questions that can Assess Suicidal Intent and Lethality in Individuals who have Attempted Suicide

- Can you describe what happened (e.g. circumstances, precipitants, view of the future, the use of alcohol or other substances, method, intent, and seriousness of injury)?
- What thoughts led up to the attempt?
- What did you think would happen (e.g. going to sleep, suffering an injury or dying, or getting a reaction out of a particular person)?
- Were other people present at the time?
- Afterwards, did you seek help yourself or did someone get help for you?
- Had you planned to be discovered or were you found accidentally?
- How did you feel afterwards (e.g. relief or regret at being alive)?
- Did you receive treatment afterwards (e.g. medical or psychiatric, emergency department, inpatient or outpatient)?
- Has your view of things changed or is anything different for you since the attempt?

Source: APA guidelines (Jacobs *et al.* 2003)

MANAGING THE PATIENT

The immediate objectives of treatment while managing a patient who displays suicidal behaviors are to (i) protect the patient from self-abuse until the suicide crisis has passed; (ii) anticipate and treat the medical complications of a suicide attempt; (iii) define and solve, if possible, the acute problem that precipitated the crisis; and (iv) diagnose and arrange treatment for the underlying problem predisposing the patient to suicidal behavior (v) deal with the acute grief reactions of the bereaved family members of suicide victims (Buzan and Weissberg 1992). Figure 8.1 represents a simple algorithm for management of individuals displaying suicidal behavior.

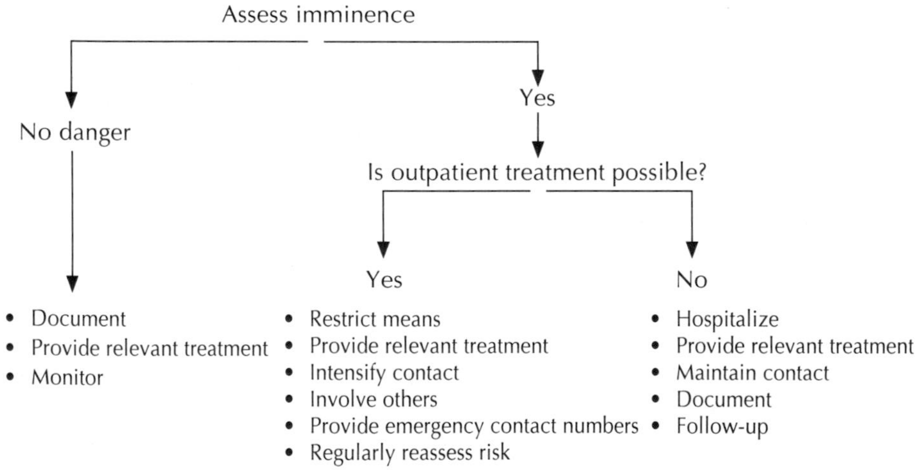

Figure 8.1 Simple algorithm for the management of individuals displaying suicidal behavior

TABLE 8.3

Checklist to Determine the Degree of Suicidal Risk

	Lower risk	Medium risk	High risk
Suicide plan			
Details	Vague	Some specifics	Clear
Availability of means	Not available	Available, has access to them close by	Has them in hand
Time	No specific time	Within a few hours	Immediately
Lethality of method	Pills, slashing wrists	Drugs and alcohol	Gun/hanging/pesticides
Chance of intervention	Others present most of the time	Others available if called upon	No one nearby, isolated
Previous suicide attempts	None or one of low lethality	Multiple of low lethality or one of medium lethality	One of high lethality or multiple of moderate lethality
Stress	None	Moderate	Severe
Symptoms			
Coping behavior	Daily activities continue as usual with little change	Some daily activities disrupted	Gross disturbances in daily functioning
Depression	Mild	Moderate	Severe
Resources	Help available	Help available but inconsistent	Help unavailable or a hostile environment
Communication aspects	Direct expression of feelings and suicidal behavior	Interpersonalized suicide goal ("They'll be sorry – I'll show them")	Very indirect or non-verbal expression of internalized suicide goal (guilt, worthlessness)
Personal life	Stable relationships and personality	Acute but short-term or psychosomatic illness	Chronic debilitating or acute catastrophic illness
Medical status	No significant medical problems	Acute but short-term or psychosomatic illness	Chronic debilitating or acute catastrophic illness

Source: Dallas Independent School District Suicide Risk Assessment Worksheet (Smith 1998)

Initial Management (Ensuring Safety and Security)

Providing safety and security should be the first step in treating the acutely suicidal patient. Some patients require admission and inpatient management. It may be

TABLE 8.4

Considerations Involved in Whether to Hospitalize the Suicidal Patient

Strongly consider hospitalization	May consider outpatient management
• Prior attempt of high lethality	• No history of potentially lethal attempts
• Well-thought-out plan	• Lack of plan/intent; cooperative family member or other adult
• Access to lethal means	• Removal or lack of availability of lethal means
• Uncommunicative	• Communicative
• Recent major loss	• Availability of intensive outpatient care
• Social isolation	• Good social support
• Hopelessness	• Hopefulness
• History of impulsive, high-risk behavior	
• Active substance abuse or dependence	
• Untreated mood, psychotic, or personality disorder	

Source: Nicholas and Golden 2001

necessary to commit the patient to a secure facility against their wishes, through legal means, if they are incompetent or refuse voluntary admission. It is important for clinicians to be aware of the legal requirements regarding involuntary commitment in the jurisdiction in which they practise (Kutcher and Chehil 2007).

As for patients who have made an unsuccessful attempt at suicide, some may require hospitalization. The factors that should be considered before admission include individual factors, the patient's support system, their living arrangements, and the feasibility and safety of other alternatives, such as intensive outpatient treatment (Table 8.4) (Nicholas and Golden 2001).

Important precautions and actions to ensure the patient's safety and security include: (i) restricting access to means of self-harm (removing potentially lethal objects, such as scissors, needles, and pesticides, from the area immediately around the patient; removing objects that one can use to hang themselves; preventing the patient from jumping out of the window or down open stairwells), (ii) constant observation and monitoring by responsible staff, (iii) anticipating and managing the medical consequences of a suicide attempt, and (iv) daily reassessment of the patient's risk of committing suicide, and deciding on the individual's level of activity and freedom of movement on the basis of the level of risk of suicide.

Suicide by ingesting pesticides is common in developing countries of South Asia. Clinicians in these countries should, therefore, possess knowledge of how to manage pesticide poisoning, particularly in rural areas, which may lack tertiary hospitals and ventilators. If the patient is conscious, activated charcoal can be given. Intravenous administration of atropine (2–4 mg in adults and 0.05–0.1 mg/kg in children every 15 minutes till atropinization is achieved) should be started if signs of cholinergic poisoning develop. If the patient develops seizures, intravenous administration of diazepam should be considered. Oral fluids and forced emesis are not recommended.

If after the assessment process, hospitalization is not deemed necessary, one can consider continuing treatment on an outpatient basis. In many cases, involvement of the family or significant others might be necessary, even if it means breaking the confidentiality clause, as the patient's safety takes precedence over confidentiality.

"No Suicide Contracts"

A "no suicide contract" is a clinical contract and not a legal one. It is an agreement, usually written, between a patient and a clinician, whereby the patient gives an undertaking that they will not harm themselves. The patient provides a "guarantee of safety", along with a "promise" to call specified individuals if there is an increase in suicidal ideation. The negotiation process must involve discussion of several aspects that are relevant to preventing the patient from committing suicide (Bertolote, de Mello-Santos and Botega 2010). The contract is based on the principle that the patient will respect the promise made to the physician. However, such a contract should never be a substitute for an informed clinical judgment based on a systematic assessment of risk. It is not recommended for agitated, psychotic, impulsive, intoxicated, and cognitively impaired patients or for adolescents.

Safety Plan

The goal of a safety plan is to empower persons in situations that have the potential to precipitate a crisis and to help them manage such situations. This is done by developing an explicit, tailored, graded, and simple series of activities to be performed by the patient when they feel distressed and suicidal. The safety plan should be developed before the patient leaves the clinic. The plan should be personalized to suit the requirements of each person. The details of the individualized safety plan, along with the relevant phone numbers, can be written on a small card which the patient can carry with them.

The safety plan basically consists of a sequenced set of instructions, including the following:

- Identify the source of the low mood (identify the behavior in advance). Engage in activities that make you feel better or distract you (e.g. go for a walk, go to the cinema, call a friend, and/or play music).
- If the suicidal thoughts continue, call (i) a support person (previously identified), (ii) a physician or mental health professional, (iii) a suicide hotline (if one is available, the number should be provided to the patient), or (iv) emergency services.

Physical Treatment

Underlying psychiatric disorders should be treated aggressively, always bearing in mind the therapeutic margin of the psychotropic agent prescribed (Nicholas and Golden 2001). Prescribing medications to suicidal patients is always a cause for concern as there is a fear that the drugs might be used to attempt suicide. However, if the signs and symptoms warrant the use of medications, the patient should not be denied the benefits of medication (Goldney 2002). Antidepressants are necessary for the treatment of depressive patients. Electroconvulsive therapy is also recommended if rapid results are required, as in the case of patients at high risk of suicide. Mood stabilizers and antipsychotic medication are useful in the treatment of bipolar patients and those with psychotic depression. Lithium is also recommended for use in patients with a high risk of suicide independent of any specific diagnosis (Raja 2009). In patients with schizophrenia and schizoaffective disorder, clozapine has been proven to be effective in reducing attempts at and completion of suicide.

Recently, ketamine (as a single bolus or intravenous infusion) has been found to be useful in emergency departments to reduce acute suicidal ideation/cognition (Kashani *et al.* 2014).

CONCLUSION

Suicidal behavior is the commonest emergency faced by psychiatrists. Handling suicidal patients is also the most anxiety-provoking situation for mental health professionals. In LAMI countries, the paucity of resources and support for clinicians during emergencies adds to the difficulties of mental health professionals. It is crucial for clinicians in developing countries to develop the competence to handle suicidal crises and attempts at suicide.

REFERENCES

Bertolote, JM and Fleischmann, A 2009, A global perspective on the magnitude of suicide mortality. In: Wasserman, D, Wasserman, C (eds). *Oxford textbook of suicidology and suicide prevention*, pp. 91–98. Oxford: Oxford University Press.

Bertolote, JM, de Mello-Santos, C and Botega, NJ 2010, Detecting suicide risk at psychiatric emergency services. *Rev Bras Psiquiatr,* 32 (Suppl 2), S87–S95.

Bryan, CJ and Rudd, MD 2006, Advances in the assessment of suicide risk. *J Clin Psychol,* 62, 185–200.

Buzan, RD and Weissberg, MP 1992, Suicide: Risk factors and therapeutic considerations in the emergency department. *J Emerg Med,* 10, 335–343.

Goldney, RD 2002, A global view of suicidal behaviour. *Emerg Med (Fremantle),* 14, 24–34.

Granello, DH 2010, The process of suicide risk assessment: Twelve core principles. *J Couns Dev,* 88, 363–371.

Harriss, L, Hawton, K and Zahl D 2005, Value of measuring suicidal intent in the assessment of people attending hospital following self-poisoning or self-injury. *Br J Psychiatry,* 186, 60–66.

Jacobs, DG, Baldessarini, RS, Conwell, Y, *et al.* 2003, Practise guideline for the assessment and treatment of patients with suicidal behaviors. In: Practice guidelines for the treatment of psychiatric disorders, *American Psychiatric Association,* 160 (11 Suppl):1–60.

Kashani, P, Yousefian, S, Amini, A, Heidari, K, Younesian, S and Hatamabadi, HR 2014, Effect of intravenous Ketamine in emergency department patients. *Emerg (Tehran),* 2, 36–39.

Krug, EG, Mercy, JA, Dahlberg, LL and Zwi, AB 2002, The world report on violence and health. *Lancet,* 360, 1083–1088.

Kutcher, S and Chehil, S 2007, Suicide intervention. In: *Suicide risk management. A manual for health professionals*, pp. 88–93. Oxford: Blackwell Publishing.

Nicholas, LM and Golden, RN 2001, Managing the suicidal patient. *Clin Cornerstone,* 3, 47–54.

Pajonk, FG, Biberthaler, P, Cordes, O and Moecke, HP 1998, Psychiatric emergencies from the viewpoint of the emergency physician. *Anaesthesist,* 47, 588–594.

Pajonk, FG, Gruenberg, KA, Moecke, H and Naber, D 2002, Suicides and suicide attempts in emergency medicine. *Crisis,* 23, 68–73.

Patton, GC, Coffey, C, Sawyer, SM, Viner, RM, Haller, DM, Bose, K, Vos, T, Ferguson, J and Mathers, CD 2009, Global patterns of mortality in young people: A systematic analysis of population health data. *Lancet,* 374, 881–892.

Raja, M 2009, Management of suicide risk in the psychiatric emergency department. In: Tatarelli, R, Pompili, M and Girardi, P (eds). *Suicide in psychiatric disorders*, pp. 99–119. New York: Nova Science Publishers.

Rockville, MD 2001, National strategy for suicide prevention: Goals and objectives for action. US Department of Health and Human Service – Public Health Service.

Rudd, MD, Berman, AL, Joiner, TE Jr, Nock, MK, Silverman, MM, Mandrusiak, M, Van Orden, K and Witte, T 2006, Warning signs for suicide: Theory, research, and clinical applications. *Suicide Life Threat Behav,* 36, 255–262.

Shneidman, ES 1985, *Definition of suicide*. New York: Wiley.

Smith, J 1998, Suicide risk assessment worksheet. Dallas Independent School District (Unpublished material): Dallas.

World Health Organization (WHO) 2014, Preventing suicide: A global imperative. Geneva, Switzerland: WHO.

9 Psychiatric Emergencies in Disaster Situations

Athula Sumathipala

INTRODUCTION

Disasters

Disasters are extraordinary events that cause destruction, death, displacement, disappearance, and disarray (Sumathipala *et al.* 2010). All of these have serious and considerable implications for those who survive. There can be varying degrees of legitimate distress arising out of this extraordinary experience. It is very unlikely that anyone who faces a disaster remains emotionally unaffected by the experience. Hence, for most, there will invariably be psychological and behavioral implications that will have an impact on their day-to-day life. However, the majority will go through the adverse experience without medium- or long-term overwhelming psychological consequences and will come to terms with their losses over a variable period of time. Therefore, it is crucial to understand the normal reaction to an extraordinary event such as a disaster.

Normal stress reactions can be behavioral, cognitive, emotional, and physical (Sumathipala *et al.* 2006).

Behavioral Reactions (Sumathipala et al. 2006)

- Sleep disorders
- Crying easily
- Avoiding reminders of the event such as holding discussions or going to those places
- Excessive activity
- Increased conflicts with the family
- Hypervigilance and startle reactions
- Isolation or social withdrawal

Cognitive Reactions (Sumathipala et al. 2006)

- Confusion and disorientation
- Intrusion of thoughts/images of the event
- Recurring dreams or nightmares
- Preoccupation with disaster
- Trouble in concentrating or difficulty in remembering

- Difficulty in making decisions
- Questioning spiritual beliefs
- Self-doubt
- Self-blame

Emotional Reactions (Sumathipala et al. 2006)

- Sadness
- Irritability, anger, and resentment
- Anxiety and fear
- Despair and hopelessness
- Guilt (survival guilt)
- Unpredictable mood swings

Physical Reactions (Sumathipala et al. 2006)

- Fatigue, exhaustion
- Gastrointestinal distress
- Change in appetite
- Tightening of the throat, chest or stomach, headache, and many other medically unexplained symptoms

It is also important to clearly understand the normal grief reactions resulting from death and other losses (Clark 2004). Grief reaction is a normal response to any loss. Feeling extremely sad, lost, guilty, crying, withdrawing from others, and not enjoying what they used to enjoy are some of the featured reactions to loss. During the immediate few weeks, every time they think of the person who died, they feel sad, and may express this by crying. These feelings may be very intense, and for most may not go away even with time. However, after a period of time, whenever they think of the deceased, they may not cry. This means that, with time, thoughts and memories get de-linked. However, if all or some of these symptoms persist for many months or even years, then it is considered as a departure from the norm. These may indicate the symptoms of unresolved or partially resolved grief.

Depression is very similar to a period of grief. Almost all of the features of grief may be seen in depression too. One should be cautious in not rushing to diagnose depression, especially if there have been no such episodes in the past. Just as physical trauma to the body evokes inflammatory responses, such as redness, swelling, heat, and pain, psychological trauma of loss leads to a sequence of natural experiences.

During phase I of grief reaction, there is shock and protest, which include numbness, disbelief, and acute dysphoria. During phase II, there is preoccupation that includes yearning, searching, and anger. Disorganization is observed in phase III, which includes despair and acceptance of loss. Finally, there is resolution in phase IV (Clark 2004).

Grief may be avoided, exaggerated, or prolonged. How grief is expressed and the rituals followed in different societies may also vary. A certain percentage of people experience a disproportionate amount of distress or grief during or in the immediate aftermath of the disaster, which may have a significant but short-term psychological and behavioral impact on their day-to-day lives and functioning. They may need urgent intervention, but this should not be necessarily considered as a psychiatric emergency (Clark 2004). However, some people with underlying predisposing factors are vulnerable, in whom the disaster can act as a precipitant and they may become mentally ill (Clark 2004). A proportion of those who are mentally ill may present as psychiatric emergencies needing urgent intervention. Such psychiatric emergencies in disaster situations can be either a new episode or a relapse of an existing illness, which may even have been in full remission. New episodes can range from an acute stress reaction to full-blown psychosis.

Relapse of an existing psychiatric condition may range from an acute panic attack to a severe psychotic episode with or without suicidal risk.

What are Emergencies?

Emergency is defined in the Oxford dictionary as "a sudden state of danger requiring immediate action and in the case of a patient a condition requiring immediate treatment" (The Oxford English Dictionary 2012). This definition implies that without such treatment, the patient's life is threatened. This is equally applicable for physical as well as psychiatric illnesses. However, in the case of a psychiatric emergency, there is a crucial difference from physical illness in terms of the risk to the patient as well as the risk to others; these include suicidal and homicidal risk.

What are the potential psychiatric emergencies? These include all those emergencies that could also be seen in non-disaster situations. The basic and core management principles are similar for all conditions and are therefore described first. Thereafter, guidelines for management are discussed.

New Acute Episodes

- A severe and extreme acute stress reaction due to loss of human life or property may even lead to suicidal ideation or suicide attempt
- Severe anxiety episode including panic
- Phobia
- Histrionic behavior
- Medically unexplained symptoms
- Psychotic episode
- Depressive episode
- Alcohol withdrawal.

Severe and Extreme Acute Stress Reactions

- A severe and extreme acute stress reaction due to loss of human life or property, leading to suicidal ideation or attempt

Acute stress reaction is a diagnosis given immediately following the experience of an exceptional mental or physical stressor.

Following a disaster, a large proportion of people may experience an 'acute trauma reaction', which is a normal reaction to the exceptional stressful situation. These symptoms could range from fear, worry, crying spells, despondency, low mood, hopelessness, suspiciousness, arousal with startle responses and even suicidal ideas. Affected persons may avoid going to the affected area or talking about the event. Most of these symptoms are seen in post-traumatic stress disorder (PTSD) but all these are common manifestations of a normal trauma reaction as well in the immediate aftermath of a disaster. Therefore, practitioners and disaster workers should be extremely cautious to not label such people as having PTSD, certainly within the first 2–3 weeks of the disaster.

International Classification of Disease (ICD-10) criteria for PTSD are (WHO 1992):

1. The patient must have been exposed to a stressful event or situation (either short or long lasting) of exceptionally threatening or catastrophic nature, which would likely cause pervasive distress in almost anyone.
2. There must be persistent remembering or reliving of the stressor in intrusive flashbacks, vivid memories or recurring dreams, or in experiencing distress when exposed to circumstances resembling or associated with the stressor.
3. The patient must exhibit an actual or preferred avoidance of circumstances resembling or associated with the stressor.
4. Either of the following must be present:
   Inability to recall either partially or completely some important aspect of the period of exposure to the stressor, OR

   Persistent symptoms of increased psychological sensitivity and arousal shown by any two of the following:

- Difficulty falling or staying asleep
- Irritability or outbursts of anger
- Difficulty in concentrating
- Hypervigilance
- Exaggerated startle response

Criteria 2, 3, and 4 must all arise within 6 months of the period of stress. The diagnostic guidelines show that the disorder should only be diagnosed after 6 months, if the symptoms are typical and do not constitute one of the other psychiatric diagnoses, such as phobic conditions, other anxiety disorders, and depression.

Therefore, PTSD should not be considered as a psychiatric emergency. Even after 6 months, diagnosing PTSD has met with severe criticism by some, and there is controversy on the diagnosis and its overuse (Summerfield 2001).

Suicide is high among those with acute stress reaction compared with those without this diagnosis, and can even be 10-fold higher (Gradus *et al.* 2010).

5. *Severe anxiety including panic*
   Anxiety and phobic symptoms are not uncommon or unusual during the immediate aftermath of a disaster. However, severe forms of these may also occur but they are uncommon.

These may be witnessed within hours of the disaster. Symptoms will include hyperventilation, shakiness, sweating, unsteadiness, and pounding of the heart. It is an extremely important clinical condition as one needs to differentiate it from acute alcohol withdrawal, which is a life-threatening medical emergency if missed. These two disorders are discussed further in Chapter 1.

6. *Medically unexplained symptoms*
   Numerous studies confirm a link between natural disasters and medically unexplained symptoms (Davidson *et al.* 1991; Escobar *et al.* 1992). A consensus statement about unexplained symptoms after terrorism and war has reiterated the importance of recognizing and managing these symptoms. During the immediate aftermath, increased reporting of physical symptoms is common (Clauw *et al.* 2003); these may simulate medical emergencies such as a heart attack (Sumathipala *et al.* 2006).
7. *A psychotic episode*
   Any psychotic symptom may manifest in people who did not previously have a known episode of psychosis. This could be acute and severe in intensity, needing immediate intervention. As the symptoms are described in Chapter 3, they will not be repeated here.
8. *A depressive episode*
   A mild, moderate, or severe depressive episode may occur but will generally manifest slowly as compared to an acute psychotic episode. In terms of management, it is considered as an emergency if the episode of depression results in disinterest in eating or drinking, leading to dehydration, severe self-neglect, and/or suicidal ideation or attempt.
9. Alcohol withdrawal is an important condition that should be detected following a disaster, as the availability of alcohol may be scarce. Those dependent on alcohol can go into a withdrawal state, which can lead to a medical emergency. It may also be misdiagnosed as a psychiatric emergency; severe acute panic, sub-acute confusional state with paranoia, and visual hallucinations (Sumathipala *et al.* 2006). Symptoms common to both panic and alcohol withdrawal include the following (Sumathipala *et al.* 2006):
   - Tremor
   - Nausea and vomiting
   - Increased sweating
   - Agitation and anxiety; mood disturbance
   - Headache
   - Hyperacusis
   - Tinnitus
   - Itching
   - Muscle cramps
   - Visual and auditory hallucinations: Many patients who are not disoriented, and who therefore do not have delirium tremens (DT), have hallucinations.

The following signs point to DT, which should be managed in a hospital. Important signs and symptoms include tachycardia, hypertension, raised body temperature, and delirium. DT is a life-threatening medical emergency. Therefore, a person who is physically dependent on alcohol should never be asked to give up drinking without supportive medical treatment.

Relapse

Relapse of all existing psychiatric illnesses among those who are under treatment is possible due to total breakdown of services and resulting non-compliance or non-availability of the treatment. The common possibilities are: (i) a psychotic episode, (ii) severe anxiety including panic, and (iii) depressive episode.

MANAGEMENT

Overall Management

Irrespective of the underlying diagnoses, management is complicated by the fact that during disasters there may be total or partial breakdown of established infrastructure, including any capacity that may have existed earlier. All those providing relief work should be mindful of this fact and should be realistic in planning management.

The overall management of a person with mental illness should be planned as given in Table 9.1.

Physical, Psychological, and Social Interventions

In psychoses, antipsychotic medication is the mainstay of treatment. Medication can reduce symptoms in around 2–4 weeks. If you start medication, it is crucial to note all the symptoms carefully in detail as the specialist would wish to re-evaluate the condition. Document the details of a delusion verbatim rather than just noting that the patient had a delusion, as at times your interpretation may be wrong. If you note these verbatim, they will be useful for the specialist in the secondary services.

Psychological and social interventions are important and are described in the WHO *Psychological first aid: Guide for field workers and Mental Health Gap Action*

TABLE 9.1

Planning for the Overall Management of a Person with Mental Illness

Management	Physical	Social	Psychological
Immediate	Need for medication	Decide the most suitable place of management Ensure safety	Empathy
Medium term	Continuation or change of medication	Social support	Psychological education Learning to deal with negative thoughts
Long term	Maintenance therapy	Re-integration with social life	Psychological education Learning to deal with negative thoughts

Programme (mhGAP) intervention guide for mental, neurological, and substance-use disorders in non-specialized health settings (WHO 2011).

Assessment, Diagnosis, and Treatment

The following are important steps in the immediate management common to all the conditions mentioned above:

- Ensuring the safety of the person by preventing suicidal attempts, which can be a major consideration irrespective of the diagnosis
- Deciding on the best place for management (home, make-shift temporary shelters vs. hospital if one exists)
- Starting medication (ideal vs. available)
- Planning on medium- to long-term management
- Engaging other relevant services

Therefore, one needs to rapidly assess the suicidal risk in every person who shows extreme distress, irrespective of whether there is an underlying psychiatric condition or an acute stress reaction.

It is important to be familiar with the comprehensive guide by WHO *Psychological first aid: Guide for field workers*. It provides a good framework for initial action (WHO 2011). There is also a WHO *Mental Health Gap Action Programme (mhGAP) intervention guide for mental, neurological, and substance-use disorders in non-specialized health settings* (WHO 2010). It presents integrated management of priority conditions using protocols for clinical decision-making. These priority conditions are depression, psychosis, bipolar disorders, epilepsy, developmental and behavioral disorders in children and adolescents, dementia, alcohol-use disorders, drug-use disorders, self-harm/suicide, and other significant emotional or medically unexplained complaints. It is a good source for managing patients in disaster settings (WHO 2010).

Where should you Manage the Person?

This is the most difficult dilemma in managing emergencies, particularly if the infrastructure is also badly damaged. Disasters and complex emergencies are defined by the breakdown of established infrastructure, including any capacity that may have existed to treat mentally ill persons. The global divide and disparities already existing within societies become wider during disasters, especially in developing countries.

Who is at High Risk?

This is an important aspect for those with both psychoses and severe depression because both these groups of patients have a high risk for suicide. Talking about suicide DOES NOT increase the risk for suicide. Therefore, if you suspect that there is a suicidal risk, never hesitate to talk about it with the person. Assessing suicidal risk is important, especially when access to care is restricted or seriously limited. Therefore, assessment of suicidal risk is an important part of the management of such patients (*see* Chapter 8).

All patients with moderate-to-severe psychoses should ideally be referred for an assessment by a psychiatrist or a medical officer for mental health or someone with experience in assessing such patients.

Indications for Urgent Referral or Need for Treatment by a Person with Greater Expertise in Mental Illness

- Moderate-to-severe suicidal risk; the risk may be higher if there was a previous attempt
- Moderate-to-severe homicidal risk (not common but possible)
- No one else is present to ensure safety
- Those who are unlikely to comply with medication
- Not eating or drinking at the time of presentation
- Coexisting psychoses
- Coexisting depression
- Poor insight or lack of it
- Self-neglect

Specific Management

Which Medication to Prescribe?

The choice of treatment depends on the availability, side-effects, and costs. There are standard local and international guidelines. Medication should be prescribed by a qualified person only, particularly if starting for the first time (Sumathipala *et al*. 2009). In limited-resource settings, the choice will depend on the availability of medications.

General Rules for Prescribing Medication

The clinical practice guidelines issued by the National Institute for Health and Care Excellence (NICE) (2015) are a valuable resource for the treatment of these conditions. The British National Formulary is also an excellent resource for prescribing medication (British Medical Association and Royal Pharmaceutical Society 2011). Guidelines by NICE recommend a generic selective serotonin reuptake inhibitor (SSRI) as the first line of treatment. However, this may not be an option in your setting. Patients should be informed about the common side-effects and withdrawal effects of the medication. Medication should be given in correct dose for at least 6 weeks before concluding that it is not effective. Medicines should be prescribed and adjusted in consultation with specialist services.

Tricyclics have more cardiotoxic effects and should be considered in case of high suicide-risk patients. Typical and atypical antipsychotic drugs should not be prescribed concurrently, except for short periods during crossover.

Antidepressants

The first line of treatment may vary between the ideal and the available antidepressant. There is no scientific evidence to suggest that one particular class of antidepressants is more efficacious than the other, although their side-effect profile may differ. This may lead to individual preferences.

Antipsychotics

The first line of treatment may vary between the ideal and available antipsychotic. The general principle is that the lowest possible dose known to be effective should be prescribed. The dose should be increased only after 2 weeks. It is good practice to use only one antipsychotic.

During the acute phase of psychoses, antipsychotic medication is necessary. There are two main classes of medication that can be used, a conventional antipsychotic and an atypical antipsychotic. In an ideal situation, an atypical antipsychotic would be the drug of choice as it has fewer short- and long-term side-effects. However, in resource-poor settings, this may not be realistic. In terms of effectiveness, chlorpromazine is no less effective than atypical antipsychotic drugs.

In case of extrapyramidal side-effects, anti-muscuranic drugs should be used such as orphenadrine hydrochloride, or procyclidine hydrochloride. However, these should not be routinely prescribed even with typical antipsychotics. These are rarely needed with atypical antipsychotics.

Duration of Treatment

First episode – continue the medication for 4–6 months after the resolution of symptoms. Therefore, the total duration is around 9 months. If medication is not continued for this period, the patient may relapse. In cases of more than one episode, the patient should be treated for at least 2 years.

Antidepressants are not addictive and there are no long-term side-effects.

Important: Every patient on an antidepressant should be monitored for signs of hyponatremia (dizziness, lethargy, confusion, cramps, and seizures). Serum sodium should be tested at baseline, 2 and 4 weeks, and after every 3 months. In case of hyponatremia, refer to a physician.

REFERENCES

British Medical Association and Royal Pharmaceutical Society 2011, British National Formulary. London: British Medical Journal Publishing Group and Pharmaceutical Press; 2011. Available at http://www.bnf.org/bnf/org_450080.htm.

Clark, A 2004, Working with grieving adults. *Advances in Psychiatric Treatment,* 10, 164–170.

Clauw, DJ, Engel, CC Jr, Aronowitz, R, Jones, E, Kipen, HM, Kroenke, K, Ratzan, S, Sharpe, M and Wessely, S 2003, Unexplained symptoms after terrorism and war: An expert consensus statement [Editorial]. *J Occup Environ Med,* 45, 1040–1048.

Davidson, JR, Hughes, D, Blazer, DG and George, LK 1991, Post-traumatic stress disorder in the community: An epidemiological study. *Psychol Med,* 21, 713–721.

Escobar, JI, Canino, G, Rubio-Stipec, M and Bravo, M 1992, Somatic symptoms after a natural disaster: Prospective study. *Am J Psychiatry,* 149, 965–967.

Gradus, JL, Qin, P, Lincoln, AK, Miller, M, Lawler, E, Sørensen, HT and Lash, TL 2010, Acute stress reaction and completed suicide. *Int J Epidemiol,* 39, 1478–1484.

National Institute for Health and Care Excellence 2015, Depression in children and young people: Identification and management. Available at http://www.nice.org.uk/guidance/published?type=cg&title=depression.

Sumathipala, A, Siribaddana, S, Mangava, S, *et al.* 2006, Cognitive behavioural therapy for medically unexplained symptoms. Colombo: Forum for Research and Development Publication.

Sumathipala, A, Siribaddana, S, Samaraweera, S, *et al.* 2009, Psychosis, severe depression, medically unexplained symptoms (MUS), epilepsy and heavy alcohol use: Identification, treatment and referral. Battramulla, Sri Lanka: Institute for Research and Development.

Sumathipala, A, Jafarey, A, De Castro, LD, Ahmad, A, Marcer, D, Srinivasan, S, Kumar, N, Siribaddana, S, Sutaryo, S, Bhan, A, Waidyaratne, D, Beneragama, S, Jayasekera, C, Edirisingha, S and Siriwardhana, C 2010, Ethical issues in post-disaster clinical interventions and research: A developing world perspective. Key findings from a drafting and consensus generation meeting of the working group on disaster research and ethics (WGDRE) 2007. *Asian Bioethics Review,* 2.2, 124–142.

Summerfield, D 2001, The invention of post-traumatic stress disorder and the social usefulness of a psychiatric category. *BMJ,* 322, 94–95.

The Oxford English Dictionary 2012. Oxford: Oxford University Press.

World Health Organization (WHO) 1992, ICD-10 classification of mental and behavioural disorders: Clinical descriptions and diagnostic guidelines. Geneva: WHO.

World Health Organization (WHO) 2010, mhGAP intervention guide for mental, neurological and substance use disorders in non-specialized health settings. Geneva: WHO. Available at http://www.who.int/mental_health/evidence/mhGAP_intervention_guide/en/index.html.

World Health Organization (WHO) 2011, Psychological first aid: Guide for field workers. Geneva: WHO. Available at: http://whqlibdoc.who.int/publications/2011/9789241548205_eng.pdf.

10 Child Psychiatric Emergencies

Tolulope Bella, Olurotimi Adejumo, Patricia Ibeziako, Olayinka Omigbodun

INTRODUCTION

Child psychiatric emergencies are situations in which there is a potential threat to the safety or well-being of the child and family. These emergencies are usually characterized by intense symptoms, perceived danger, a sense of urgency, and the perception of an immediate catastrophic outcome (Martin, Volmar and Lewis 2007). The functioning and well-being of children are highly dependent on their family, school, and the community in which they live. Child psychiatric emergencies usually represent some dysfunction in one or more of the elements of this delicately balanced system. They are mostly the outcome of complex, ongoing processes and a long history of emotional and behavioral difficulties rather than being sudden discrete events.

In many parts of the developing world, children live in extremely difficult social circumstances. Several children are separated from their families as a result of extended fostering and other cultural practices, disease epidemics, wars, and disasters. These situations may result in abandonment, orphanhood, children living on the streets, and in refugee camps (Department for International Development 2006). Scores of children do not attend school for reasons such as extreme poverty, violence, and social chaos. All these factors increase the vulnerability of children in these regions to psychiatric emergencies. Rarely does a child present with a psychiatric emergency without previous warning signs, as a child in crisis typically reflects a family or community system in crisis. The people who are the most likely to define a situation as an emergency are the child's parents or guardians or other adults in the environment on whom the child depends.

In the developing world, parents or guardians usually declare the child's behavior problems an emergency when they can no longer cope with the behavior, and often after consultations with trusted friends and traditional or religious healers have failed. Given the high rates of infectious diseases and poor nutrition in the developing world, many psychiatric emergencies are related to underlying general medical conditions and may occur in the form of acute organic brain syndromes. Acute organic brain syndromes often manifest with varying degrees of behavioral abnormalities, which may require urgent psychiatric intervention. In addition, the occurrence of deliberate self-harm among adolescents sometimes follows adverse psychosocial events within the personal or family context.

COMMON SITUATIONS LEADING TO CHILD AND ADOLESCENT PSYCHIATRIC EMERGENCIES IN LOW-RESOURCE SETTINGS

Generally in low-resource settings, child and adolescent psychiatric emergencies arise as a result of an exacerbation of a pre-existing psychiatric disorder, acute traumatic experiences, or from complications of a medical condition or treatment. Some examples of each of these situations are outlined below:

- Pre-existing psychiatric disorders could constitute an emergency in the event of a relapse or an exacerbation of symptoms. An adolescent with bipolar disorder could present with disruptive and physically aggressive behavior during an acute manic episode, presenting risk of harm to self, harm to others, and/or harm to property.
- Some presentations may be unrelated to prior psychiatric conditions but would require psychiatric intervention due to the child or adolescent's exposure to a traumatic situation. Traumatic situations may be a result of physical, psychological, or sexual abuse and child neglect. It is often critical to address the child's psychological state after the traumatic event. Physical and psychological abuse may arise as a complication of attempts at addressing mental health problems using non-orthodox methods such as physical incarceration, beating, and various methods for exorcism.
- Disorders such as epilepsy remain prevalent in low-resource settings. In several situations, children may present to mental health professionals with epileptic seizures. Disruptive behavioral patterns predominate in children with complex partial seizures, and other health practitioners may refer them to a psychiatrist or mental health professional.

Acute reactions to medications such as "typical" antipsychotics used more frequently in low-resource settings, may constitute a child psychiatric emergency. Children or adolescents experiencing an oculogyric crisis, tongue protrusion, torticollis, other forms of acute dystonic reaction, or akathisia may require urgent intervention by a mental health professional.

COMMON PRECIPITATING FACTORS FOR CHILD EMERGENCIES

Factors that precipitate child emergencies can be divided into individual factors, those related to the family, those related to the school, and social factors (Table 10.1). The following potential psychosocial precipitants of child emergencies were identified in a child psychiatry clinic in Ibadan, Nigeria (Omigbodun 2004):

- Problems with primary support as a result of separation, abandonment, child fostering, and the use of children for labor.
- Educational problems, such as poor academic performance, lack of appropriate school placement, discord with teachers or classmates, and removal from formal school settings.
- Prolonged fasting by a child for religious reasons.

TABLE 10.1

Precipitating Factors for Child Psychiatric Emergencies

Family factors	• Parental separation or divorce • Parental abandonment • Illness or death in the family • Poor parent–child communication
School factors	• Academic failure • Peer problems • Bullying
Individual factors	• Physical and intellectual disability • Chronic physical illness • Isolation • Impulsive behavior • Poor social skills • Broken romantic relationships
Social factors	• Socioeconomic disadvantage • Social discrimination • Isolation • Neighborhood violence

Source: Adapted from *Lewis' child and adolescent psychiatry* (Martin, Volmar and Lewis 2007)

- Keeping a child with psychiatric illness in a traditional healer's home for several years.
- The child being given "traditional treatment" (including scarification and forced ingestion of traditional concoctions) by relatives.
- Ongoing physical abuse of the child by caregivers to get rid of the "demons" responsible for psychosis or conduct problems.

SOURCES OF REFERRAL FOR CHILD EMERGENCY ASSESSMENTS

The common sources of referral for psychiatric emergencies among children in the developing world are:

- Parents and guardians
- School teachers and counselors
- Medical staff working with hospitalized children
- Family physicians or pediatricians
- Members of the extended family
- Other concerned individuals.

GOALS OF ASSESSMENT

General Principles of the Child and Parent Interview and Mental State Assessment

The overall goals of the emergency psychiatric evaluation of the child or adolescent are to first identify and manage the immediate concerns of safety, clarify the nature and cause of the imbalance in the child's ecosystem (Martin, Volmar and Lewis 2007), and identify the resources needed to restore equilibrium, such as:

- A safe environment
- Psychoeducation for the child or adolescent, family members, teachers, and other significant individuals
- Psychopharmacological interventions
- Psychotherapy
- Family support services.

Emergency Evaluation

The emergency evaluation should involve the following:

- Obtain each informant's account of the nature and reasons for the emergency.
- Obtain a developmental history that includes the current difficulties, as well as the child's prior functioning in the context of his family, school, and living situations.
- Rule out and treat underlying medical conditions.
- Develop differential diagnoses and attempt to form an idea of what precipitated the emergency.
- Arrive at a judgment of the probable risk to the safety of the child and others.
- Identify interventions that can contain or ameliorate the child's difficulties.
- Develop a working alliance with all members of the child's ecosystem.
- Plan and implement safe disposition (how and where to treat) and follow-up care.

THE PHYSICAL SETTING

In low-resource settings, the evaluation of a child in an emergency situation usually takes place in the general emergency room, pediatric ward or an outpatient clinic. The evaluation could also take place in a community setting, such as a school, primary healthcare clinic, or the juvenile justice system, as most children are unable to access specialized child psychiatry services.

The ideal environment for an emergency evaluation should have the following features:

- It should be free of sharp objects, cords, or potentially hazardous equipment.
- It should allow for privacy and not permit excessive sensory stimulation, such as from noise and excessive physical activity.
- There should be some level of visual surveillance from outside, and other staff and security personnel should be able to easily access the evaluation area.
- The place should be spacious enough to allow for seclusion or restraint, if needed (Martin, Volmar and Lewis 2007).

THE CHILD AND ADOLESCENT PSYCHIATRY INTERVIEW

Cultural practices in several parts of the developing world result in situations whereby children are not used to being heard or spoken to (Omigbodun 2008). The mental health professional thus needs to use interviewing and observational skills that will encourage the child to speak, as well as pay attention to both verbal and non-verbal cues. It is important to make attempts to interview adolescents and older children privately to encourage them to speak freely about their concerns.

- The interview of the child should take into account the child's age and developmental level. Younger children are generally less articulate.
- The child may have generated a crisis and may want to talk about it, or may be reticent or withdrawn. The child may feel forced into treatment.
- The child may also be so overwhelmed and frightened by the reaction to what they have done that they may try to minimize the problem. For example, a child who has attempted suicide by hanging may say, "I was just playing and I never wanted to die."
- It is important not to be confrontational or accusatory towards the child, no matter how bad the behavior.
- Observe how the child relates to family members, and the extent to which the child can agree on the problems to be addressed and how to address them.

MENTAL STATE EXAMINATION

During the mental state examination (Martin, Volmar and Lewis 2007), it is important to look out for the following:

- Signs of disorientation, confusion, and fluctuating levels of consciousness
- Psychomotor agitation or retardation, restlessness
- Neurological signs, such as slurred speech, ataxia, and apraxia
- Depressed or angry mood, mood lability
- Incoherence of thought and speech
- Suicidal or homicidal ideation
- Aggressive threats or ideation
- Perceptual disturbances
- Impulsivity
- Impaired memory
- Poor judgment and insight
- Limited intelligence.

PRINCIPLES OF MANAGEMENT OF CHILD PSYCHIATRIC EMERGENCIES

An emergency or crisis presents an opportunity for intervention and change, and child and adolescent mental health (CAMH) professionals should make the best use of the situation. Although making an accurate diagnosis is essential, sometimes the complaint with which the child presents has little significance for psychiatric diagnosis and management, being just a sign of the child's distress. In some instances, the crisis could be handled most effectively by managing parental psychopathology. While developing the treatment plan, health professionals should consider the biopsychosocial formulation and diagnosis of the child, parent, or other caregiver. This should inform the development of the treatment plan.

- Ensure the safety of the child and of those around, and see to it that the child is protected against self-harm or an abusive environment. At the same time, make sure the child does not pose a threat to others. Hospitalization or putting the child in a foster home is one of the best ways to ensure safety. Most resource-poor settings do not have separate treatment facilities for children and adolescents who have psychiatric illnesses and require inpatient care. This unfortunate situation may compel CAMH professionals dealing with emergency situations to admit children and adolescents in adult inpatient facilities. Social welfare services are also often poorly organized in low-resource settings, and there may be no organized foster care. However, these support roles can be fulfilled by the extended family system, which can come in very handy at such times. If a child is suicidal, depressed, psychotic, or impulsive, it may be more important to focus first on managing the urgent complaints (in terms of behavior and emotional disturbances) before exploring the underlying psychosocial issues.
- It is essential to establish communication with the child, and between the child and family.
- The child is sometimes the 'identified patient' in a family with multiple problems and must not be made a scapegoat for the problems in the family.

SPECIFIC PSYCHIATRIC EMERGENCIES IN CHILDREN

- Delirium
- Aggression, violence, psychosis
- Deliberate self-harm and attempted suicide
- Physical and sexual abuse of the child
- Drug or substance-induced problems (intoxication and adverse drug reactions)
- Conduct disorder (violence, running away from home)
- Anxiety disorders (generalized anxiety disorder [GAD], panic disorder, post-traumatic stress disorder [PTSD] with flashbacks)
- Dissociative disorders.

Delirium

Delirium occurs among critically ill children all over the world. It is a disturbance of consciousness and cognition that develops acutely, and has a fluctuating course characterized by inattention and an impaired ability to receive, process, store, or recall information. Delirium results from medical conditions, exposure to substances, medication, toxins, and multiple causes (American Psychiatric Association 2013). Pediatric delirium may be extremely subtle and may be complicated by the developmental variability in clinical presentations. It may also be associated with other neuropsychiatric symptoms, such as purposeless actions, inconsolability, and signs of autonomic dysregulation. A large retrospective study revealed that morbidity in children diagnosed with delirium is relatively high and the mortality rate is 20%

(Smith *et al.* 2009). Critical illness in the pediatric patient causes acute and chronic organ dysfunction, which may progress to long-term neurological sequelae.

Clinical Approach to Delirium

The clinical approach to preventing or treating delirium may vary and be driven by different goals, including the following:

- Control of precipitating risk factors (infection, electrolyte abnormalities, sleep deprivation, and exposure to medication or substances)
- Management of the symptoms of delirium (psychosis or agitation)
- Treatment of delirium through the resolution of the underlying cause.

Psychosocial Management

Maintaining as normal an environment as possible within the hospital setting allows for consistent orientation of the patient and helps to reassure the child (Martin, Volmar and Lewis 2007). The strategies used to deal with critically ill children with delirium include the following.

- Try to ensure the child's parents or caregivers are present.
- The child should be regularly shown pictures of familiar people and objects.
- Playing familiar music might help the child.
- A CAMH professional could be engaged for behavioral management of the child.

Delirium Medication Management

- Although medications used to manage delirium may control agitation and disruptive behavior in the short term, they have adverse psychoactive effects that may worsen a patient's sensorium and lead to prolonged cognitive impairment. Haloperidol is a conventional antipsychotic agent that is used frequently for the treatment of delirium. However, in hypoactive delirium, which is associated with dopamine depletion versus excess, treatment with haloperidol may exacerbate the severity of delirium and prolong psychomotor retardation, or even promote catatonic features.
- Atypical antipsychotic agents, such as risperidone, olanzapine, and ziprasidone, are considered alternatives to haloperidol for the treatment of delirium. The potential clinical benefits of this class of medications include their global impact on dopamine receptors, as well as their effects on serotonin, acetylcholine, and norepinephrine neurotransmission.

Agitation, Aggression, and Violence

Agitation is a presentation common to many psychiatric conditions and is considered a psychiatric emergency. The core features generally described are:

- Restlessness with excessive or semi-purposeful motor activity
- Irritability
- Heightened responsiveness to internal and external stimuli
- An unstable course.

TABLE 10.2

Causes of Aggression in Children and Adolescents

Younger children	Adolescents
Reaction to interpersonal conflicts and difficulties in their environment (inconsistent or abusive parenting, lack of appropriate discipline)	Bipolar disorder
Psychosis	Depression
Severe ADHD (attention deficit hyperactivity disorder)	Substance abuse/ reaction
Seizure disorder	Schizophrenia

Source: Adapted from *Lewis' child and adolescent psychiatry* (Martin, Volmar and Lewis 2007)

Note that aggression is not always associated with agitation, and the frequency with which agitation is associated with aggression is not known. The features disposing an individual to make the transition from simple agitation to aggression are poorly understood (Nordstrom and Allen 2007). Aggression and violence in youth may reflect biological factors, such as psychosis and delirium, as well as psychosocial factors including a child's reaction to interpersonal conflict and threats in his or her environment (Table 10.2).

Management of Aggression in Youth

- Aggressive or agitated adolescents should first be managed with the "talking down" approach, verbal redirection, and behavioral interventions. Youth should also be gently offered assistance and support.
- If the above methods prove unsuccessful, chemical restraint (medications) should be considered for the next line of management.
- Physical restraints should be used only when less restrictive methods have failed and there is imminent danger to the safety of the child or adolescent, or that of others.
- The use of physical restraints should be discontinued once the patient's behavior is under control and the danger has passed.
- Ideally, during the period when physical restraints are being used, the child or adolescent should be monitored for restriction of the airway, changes in the breathing pattern, reduced circulation, or changes in body temperature. Such monitoring, however, remains a challenge in the parts of the developing world because of the severe shortage of trained CAMH professionals.

Emergency Pharmacotherapy for Aggressive Youth

The pharmacologic treatment of aggression in children and adolescents has presented some controversy for clinicians and researchers over the years, partly due to a paucity of evidence for efficacy versus risk for various agents used in adults. Additional challenges exist in low-resource settings where several pharmacologic agents are not available, and where adverse socioeconomic realities may limit patient access to available agents. In many of these low-resource settings, healthcare is financed by out-of-pocket payment. It has been recommended that the ideal pharmacologic agent for chemical restraint should have a number of characteristics, including (i) established efficacy in childhood, (ii) multiple routes of administration, (iii) not induce dependence or tolerance, (iv) have minimal side-effects, and (v) be cost-effective (Sorrentino 2004). Although no single medication is known to meet all of these criteria, a number of medicines have been employed in the management of aggression in youth. These are briefly discussed below.

- First-generation antipsychotic agents, such as haloperidol and chlorpromazine, are the most readily available drugs in the developing world. The method of administration in an emergency depends on the severity of the target symptoms, the cooperation of the child, and the drug formulations available. The oral route is the preferred method as it is less invasive and allows affected children to participate in exerting some control over their behavior. Liquid preparations are preferable to pills as they cannot be hidden in the child's mouth, and absorption is thus better guaranteed. Unfortunately, liquid formulations of these agents are generally not available in many low-resource settings. The intramuscular route may be used when a faster onset of action is required and the patient is uncooperative with oral or intravenous administration. Haloperidol can be given both orally and parenterally.

BOX 10.1

KY, an 11-year-old girl, presented to the infectious disease clinic of the University College Hospital, Ibadan with a 5-year history of swelling of the neck, recurrent cough, and blood-stained sputum. She had been receiving treatment from a traditional healer in her village who had excised some of the swellings. She was the only surviving child of her parents, who had died 3 years earlier following a diagnosis of tuberculosis (TB) and acquired immune deficiency syndrome (AIDS). Her younger sibling had also died a few years earlier. After the death of her parents, she dropped out of school and had been living with her grandmother. She moved in with an uncle a few weeks before visiting the hospital.

She was diagnosed with stage 4 HIV infection and infection with disseminated TB. Appropriate treatment was commenced. While admitted in hospital, she had repeated altercations with other patients in the ward. During one of the altercations, she bit another child's hand, the wound being a deep one. The incident resulted in an emergency referral to the child psychiatrist.

Psychiatric evaluation revealed the presence of anxiety, anger, and worry about her illness and her future, as well as unresolved grief related to the death of her family members. She received supportive therapy and grief counseling. The patient was also introduced to basic interpersonal skills. She had a total of four sessions and no further outbursts of aggressive behavior were reported (Oladokun *et al*. 2008).

Parenteral administration of chlorpromazine is not advocated for children because it is associated with a risk of postural hypotension even at very low doses.

- Second-generation antipsychotics are generally less freely available in most parts of the developing world, compared to better-resourced settings. Oral risperidone is however available in many parts of the developing world. Olanzapine is available in some regions, both in the oral and fast-acting intramuscular formulations. Two placebo-controlled studies comparing intramuscular olanzapine to intramuscular haloperidol showed that both had a similar efficacy at 2 hours and 24 hours after the first dose. Both studies found that olanzapine was better tolerated, and haloperidol was more likely to cause adverse events such as acute dystonia and medication-induced Parkinsonism (Nordstrom and Allen 2007). The concurrent use of intramuscular olanzapine and intramuscular/intravenous benzodiazepines is not recommended as fatalities from respiratory depression have been reported in adults, although causality is yet to be firmly established (Marder *et al.* 2010). Aripiprazole is not widely available in most parts of the developing world. Haloperidol is the only medication currently considered a first-line agent for medical (organic) conditions.
- Benzodiazepines can also be used to control aggression. However, they must be avoided in cases in which the use of other drugs is suspected, and especially in disorders where there is depression of the central nervous system, due to the risk of drug interactions and respiratory depression. Only oral formulations of benzodiazepines, such as lorazepam, are currently approved for children.
- The use of oral antihistamines (e.g. diphenhydramine) is widespread in emergency rooms in well-resourced settings. The purpose is to sedate the patient (although there is not much evidence to support their efficacy). Antihistamines are also used in conjunction with antipsychotics to prevent extrapyramidal side-effects (Scivoletto, Boarati and Turkiewicz 2010).
- The use of other medications depends on the specific diagnosis (e.g. seizures, psychosis, and conduct disorder).

Deliberate Self-harm and Attempted Suicide

Suicidal behavior in youth is recognized as an important health and social problem, and is now among the top five causes of death among young people worldwide. It is one of the leading causes of emergency referrals all over the world, although less common among pre-adolescents than adolescents. Deciphering the behavior of a child who has the intent to cause self-harm can be challenging. Young children are generally believed not to have the logic or cognitive abilities to plan, understand the consequences of, and follow through with the preparation for suicide. The method used for suicide reveals the strength of the intent, with the use of firearms, hanging and strangling indicating stronger intent than a drug overdose.

Suicide threats and behavior may reflect a cry for help and may be related to the achievement of some other goal other than self-harm. Suicidal behavior may also arise from problems with communication within the child's family. However, some children actually commit suicide. It is, therefore, important to identify those who are at an increased risk. While making an assessment, it is important to identify risk factors such

TABLE 10.3

Risk Factors for Suicide and Self-harm

Demographic factors	
Age	The risk for suicidal and self-harm in pre-pubertal children is smaller and increases during middle and older adolescence.
Gender	Males are at a greater risk of completed suicide, although girls make three times as many attempts.
Presence of depression	Major depression with accompanying symptoms of poor self-esteem, hopelessness, helplessness, loneliness, and a sense of guilt may be the most important risk factors.
Presence of conduct disorder	Anti-social males are more likely to harm themselves and others, especially if they also abuse alcohol and drugs. Impaired judgment and impulse control problems are associated with the use of drugs and can be deadly.
Previous suicide attempts	Previous attempts increase the risk of completed suicide.
Family distress and psychopathology	Stressful life events, such as disruption of the family, discord in the family, violence, and physical abuse, are important risk factors for suicidal ideation or attempts among pre-adolescent children.
School factors	Bullying at school has been found to be a risk factor for suicide.

as age, gender, the presence of depression or conduct disorder, substance use problems, a prior suicide attempt, and a family history of suicide (Table 10.3).

The past decade has seen an increase in epidemiological studies on suicidal behavior in the developing world, possibly resulting from increased reporting rates. According to a Nigerian study, over 20% of adolescents between the ages of 10 and 17 years in Ibadan, South-West Nigeria reported suicidal ideation, and approximately 12% had attempted suicide in the previous year (Omigbodun 2008). The factors that had a significant association with suicidal ideation were socioeconomic deprivation evidenced by having to go hungry due to a lack of food at home, having to earn a living, and a lack of family cohesion reflected in having separated or divorced parents. In the Zambian global school-based health study, 31.3% of adolescents reported suicidal ideation in the preceding 12 months, and worry, sadness, hopelessness, ever been drunk, and the use of marijuana were associated with suicidal ideation (Muula *et al.* 2007). Similarly, in rural Uganda, the 12-month prevalence of suicidal ideation among adolescent students was 21.6% (Rudatsikira *et al.* 2007). Being female, of relatively older age, engaging in cigarette smoking, using alcohol, having been bullied, loneliness, significant worry, and lack of parental supervision were associated with suicidal ideation. In Cote d'Ivoire, family conflicts, failure in school, and emotional difficulties have also been associated with suicidal behaviors (Yéo-Tenena *et al.* 2010). In Asia, the one-year prevalence of attempted suicide among Chinese youth was 2.7% (Xing *et al.* 2010). Separation from parents and family social problems were identified as risk factors in this population (Xing *et al.* 2010). In addition to parent and family-related factors, deliberate self-harm behaviors were associated with suicidal behavior among school-based adolescents in a more recent study (Xing, Qiao, Duan and Bai 2015). Another study found significant association between perpetration of, and victimization from cyberbullying, and suicidal behavior among Chinese high school adolescents (Wang *et al.* 2015).

In the developing world, children between the ages of 10 and 19 have been reported to use various methods to self-harm. These include ingesting poisons, taking drug overdoses, and hanging (Nigeria); ingesting chemical agents such as chloroquine and psychotropics (Abidjan, Cote d'Ivoire); hanging, ingesting poisons, and shooting (Ghana); hanging in the case of males and both hanging and poisoning in the case of females (South Africa); taking drug overdoses and ingesting pesticides (Tehran in particular); and inflicting burn injuries on oneself (Iran in general) (Yéo-Tenena *et al.* 2010; Adinkrah 2011; Burrows and Laflamme 2008; Ghazinour *et al.* 2009; Groohi *et al.* 2006).

Assessment of Suicidal Youth

The management of suicidal children and adolescents should involve an evaluation of the child's suicidal behavior and determination of the risk for death or repetition, as well as an assessment of the underlying diagnoses or promoting factors (Schaffer, Gould and Hicks 2007). The underlying diagnosis should be treated appropriately and psychosocial interventions instituted for the promoting factors.

The following should be taken into account while making an evaluation of suicidal behavior:

- The method used, including its lethality
- The youth's intent and perception of lethality
- The factors that have precipitated the attempt
- The degree of planning involved in making the attempt
- Chance of rescue
- Disclosure of the attempt
- The frequency and duration of suicidal ideation before and after the attempt.

Child Abuse

Both physical and sexual abuse can give rise to either acute or delayed emergency symptoms. The abuse may be obvious (rape, serious physical injury) or disguised (incest, moderate physical abuse, or neglect).

Epidemiology

Exposure to physical and sexual abuse is relatively poorly documented in the developing world. A global health survey carried out in five countries of east and southern Africa (Namibia, Swaziland, Uganda, Zambia, and Zimbabwe) found that the average lifetime prevalence rate of exposure to physical abuse was 42% and that of exposure to sexual abuse, 23% (Brown *et al.* 2009). Malemo Kalisya *et al.* (2011)

found that in the Democratic Republic of Congo, children and youth were more often assaulted by someone known to the family than by military personnel and more often had a delayed presentation (i.e. >72 hours) to medical services. Afifi *et al*. (2003) found that the prevalence of physical abuse among Egyptian adolescents was 7.6%, while that of sexual abuse was 7%. The significant predictors of sexual abuse were being a hyperactive child, having a disability, having a disinterested mother, being low in the birth order, or being a wasted child. For physical abuse, the significant predictors were having a disinterested mother, having a mother with a low level of education, and having injuries.

In the Ibadan adolescent health study, a mental and physical health survey of randomly selected youth in urban and rural schools in South-West Nigeria (Omigbodun 2011), it was found that the average age at which Nigerian youth were sexually abused was 8.59 years (SD 2.99) (Omigbodun 2011). Sexual abuse was reported by 13.8% of the study sample (208 out of 1,504). Of those subjected to sexual abuse, 40.9% had been abused by cousins, uncles, or aunts; 31.8% by domestic help; 4.5% by teachers; and 22.7% by neighbors. The significant predictors of sexual abuse identified for this population were:

- Rural dwelling
- Reduced parental supervision
- Suicidal symptoms
- Depressive symptoms
- Use of alcohol and nicotine.

Assessment

- Cases of abuse are identified mostly by pediatricians or family physicians, and a psychiatrist may be called upon to assess the emotional status of the patient and the family.
- Clinically, the abused child may appear frightened, evasive, and aggressive, and may adopt a defensive stance. Apathy, somnolence, and sadness are also common features.
- It is not uncommon for children to deny any history of abuse despite clear signs, due to the fear of being held responsible for a family crisis or a fear of incurring future aggression from the perpetrator.
- It is important to watch the child's verbal and non-verbal reactions in the presence of different family members. A display of more intense anxiety, fear, or aggressiveness towards a specific person could be a pointer to the perpetrator of the abuse.
- Suspicions of maltreatment or abuse must be based on the clinical history, physical examination, and diagnostic imaging examinations. The absence of indicators in the history and examinations does not exclude the possibility of abuse, in the same way that isolated findings cannot be taken as a positive indication of victimization.

Management

The role of a psychiatrist in cases of abuse is to help identify such cases or raise suspicion when such cases are brought to their knowledge; provide emergency supportive care; and communicate with the other members of the multidisciplinary team.

The management of victims of abuse should have four main objectives:

- Attempts should be made to avoid subsequent abuse by removing the child from the environment in which the abuse is taking place (this is often a challenge in resource-poor settings as there may be no available safe alternatives for the child).
- An effort must be made to provide relief for the effects of the past event, i.e. it is necessary to treat the child with understanding and provide support.
- An assessment must be made of the child's emotional, social and educational needs following the event.
- In parts of the developing world where there are no child protection services, the psychiatrist or a multidisciplinary team of psychologists, social workers, and health personnel could provide supportive counseling. As the child may be suffering from extreme guilt, health personnel should be empathic and non-judgmental and should not lay blame on the child. Even if they are not the perpetrators of the abuse, the parents of most abused children should receive appropriate psychoeducation so that they do not blame the child, but instead, offer support and protection from future abuse.

Substance Use Problems

While substance and alcohol use disorders are becoming increasingly common among the youth, acute intoxication and drug reactions are less common presentations than psychosis and aggression in low- and middle-income settings.

Assessment

- Bizarre behavior associated with confusion, coma, or respiratory or circulatory changes should raise suspicion of substance use problems.
- Urine and blood screening are necessary, but this may be a challenge in low-resource settings.
- Drug antagonists are not always available.
- Problems associated with substance use are often comorbid with other disorders, such as depression, psychosis, and environmental abuse. The final evaluation of a patient presenting with substance-related problems should include an assessment of the family, and one should wait until the intoxication and reactions to the substance or drug have resolved. Otherwise, other underlying psychopathology may be missed.

Conduct Disorder

Children with conduct problems can be particularly difficult to engage as they are often very wary of adults. All efforts should be made to resolve their acute as well as long-term problems, which are usually related to communication problems within the family.

Anxiety, Dissociative, and Somatoform Disorders

Typical anxiety crises are not very common among children in low- and middle-income countries, among whom anxiety is often manifested as somatic symptoms (e.g. headaches and abdominal pain). There may be episodes of loss of consciousness, syncope, and motor or sensory dysfunctions, resembling epileptic seizures. In these cases, it is advisable to perform a neurological examination, electroencephalography, and neuroimaging where possible. In the case of an acute anxiety crisis, patients should be properly medicated so that they obtain immediate relief from their symptoms, and also to allow for a reassessment of the episode. Low doses of benzodiazepines with a short half-life can be used, since their effect is instantaneous and they do not cause excessive somnolence (Scivoletto, Boarati and Turkiewicz 2010). Support and psychoeducation often form the mainstay of treatment in low-resource settings.

Dissociative disorders typically manifest as disruptions or a discontinuity in the normal functions of consciousness, memory, identity, emotion, perception, body representation, motor control, and behavior (American Psychiatric Association 2013). Dissociative disorders may present with "positive" symptoms such as depersonalization, derealization, or fragmentation in the experience of identity, or subjective "negative" experiences, with loss of access or control over mental functions such as memory, resulting in dissociative amnesia (American Psychiatric Association 2013). Children and adolescents who experience traumatic events, including maltreatment, abuse, natural disasters, or war are at increased risk of dissociative disorders (American Psychiatric Association 2013; Shipman and Taussig 2009; Laor *et al*. 2002; Cagiada, Candido and Pennati 1997).

Dissociative disorders manifest in a variety of ways, and the following presentations should raise suspicion of disorders in this category (International Society for the Study of Dissociation 2004):

- *Trance states or "black outs"*. These may range between transient absences of attention to longer periods of non-responsiveness, and may be as severe as to mimic a comatose state (Cagiada, Candido and Pennati 1997).
- *Amnesia and transient forgetting*. Common indicators of a dissociative process may be amnesia for past traumatic events. Children may also feign forgetfulness due to unwillingness to report trauma or abuse to an unfamiliar individual, hence it is important to show empathy in therapy and work at developing a good rapport with the child as early as possible.
- *Imaginary playmates*. Imaginary playmates may be a normal developmental phenomenon, but fantasy that interferes with normal activity, or in which the child feels their behavior is out of their control is likely to be pathological. Also, imaginary individuals perceived as real, as threatening to the child, or in conflict with each other, may be indicative of a dissociative disorder.
- *Identity alteration*. Although relatively uncommon, children may display behavior suggestive of alternative self-states or personalities.
- *Sudden changes in behavior* during the interview, such as regression, sudden rageful behavior, apparent loss of consciousness, seizure-like activity, or suddenly talking about oneself in the third person or with a new name.

- *Depersonalization or derealization.* The presence of comorbid substance use should be ruled out, especially in adolescents.
- *Somatic symptoms.* As part of assessing the child's current functioning, it is important to inquire about somatic symptoms including headaches, abdominal pain, other undiagnosed pain, or loss of physical sensations.
- *Post-traumatic symptoms.* These may include "positive" symptoms such as nightmares, night terrors, disturbing hypnagogic hallucinations, intrusive disturbing thoughts and memories, re-experiencing, or flashbacks, or "negative" symptoms such as numbing and avoidance.
- *Sexually suggestive behavior*, sexually reactive, or sexually offending behavior may be seen in traumatized children, and may occur alongside dissociative symptoms.
- *Self-injurious behavior* is reported to occur commonly as part of dissociative phenomena among adolescents, and may include cutting, burning, scratching, or head banging. This behavior may be carried out in secret and may serve an affect-regulating function. Sometimes it may occur as part of a dissociative trance state.

Assessment of Dissociative Symptoms

Assessment should involve inquiring about symptoms relating to those outlined above. It is important for the interviewer or therapist to inquire cautiously, beginning with discussing non-anxiety provoking events or experiences (such as the child's everyday activities, experiences, or favorite habits), and gradually progressing toward more potentially disturbing events or experiences. During the interview process, it is important to evaluate how the child or adolescent's symptoms interfere with normal developmental tasks. The following areas are key to assessing a child with dissociative symptoms (International Society for the Study of Dissociation 2004).

- *Clinical interview.* This should include an exploration of the child's presenting symptoms by evaluating the significance of the symptoms, and possibly the underlying trauma, of the child. The clinical interview should also involve an assessment of the family environment, particularly with respect to physical and emotional safety; dysfunctional family relationships; family history of psychiatry illness; unique beliefs, practices, or secrets held in the family; and the family's understanding of the child's symptoms. It is important to assess the child's exposure to material relevant to the dissociative symptoms, such as having witnessed such symptoms in other individuals, or exposure to relevant material from movies, books, or conversations with others. The child's functioning in other settings, especially school, and his or her interactions with peers, teachers, and others must be explored. It is important to identify perpetuating risk factors, in addition to predisposing and precipitating ones. Beyond examining possible areas of trauma in the child's past, a focus on existing stressful patterns in the family or environment is necessary to preventing maintenance of the child's symptoms.
- *Assessment of comorbidities.* As dissociative disorders are frequently comorbid with other psychiatric conditions, the child should be evaluated for post-traumatic stress symptoms, obsessive–compulsive disorder (OCD), affective disorders, substance use disorders, and specific developmental disorders.

- *Medical evaluation.* It is important to rule out existing general medical conditions that may mimic dissociative symptoms, including seizure disorders, other neurological conditions, allergic conditions, such as bronchial asthma, and legal or illegal drug effects. If found, general medical conditions may take priority over any identified psychopathology.

Management of Dissociative Disorders

An important initial step in the management of dissociative and somatoform disorders is the exclusion of organic/neurological pathophysiology through an extensive medical work-up. The resources required for this are not always available in low- and middle-income settings, where dissociative disorders are infrequently diagnosed. However, it is important for psychiatrists and mental health care workers in these settings to have a high index of suspicion when dealing with unusual presenting symptoms for which a definite medical etiology cannot be established, especially if a history of trauma cannot be elicited.

Once organic etiology has been ruled out, generally, dissociative symptoms in children and adolescents are less complicated and of shorter duration than in adult cases. An optimistic attitude by the therapist may facilitate recovery. It is important to determine early in the assessment process, how to best manage the child, considering available resources. Severe cases may require inpatient treatment, while the availability of a multidisciplinary team including community and social workers may enable care to take place outside of potentially restrictive inpatient services. The following points are important to note in the management of dissociative disorders.

- It is beneficial to ensure continuity in the therapist's relating to the child through the therapeutic process.
- Treatment is often a team effort. Even within the personnel constraints of low-resource settings, efforts should be made to establish links with the family, school, and other significant parties involved in the child's life. Communication among these parties is crucial, and the therapist should coordinate these communications to ensure a focused approach to caring for the child as he or she progresses along in treatment.
- While building an empathic relationship with the patient, the therapist must balance confidentiality with information that may have life-threatening implications. These policies should be disclosed to both the child and caregivers at the beginning of therapy.
- Treatment should include intervention with the family. At the very least, in-depth psychoeducation on the nature of the child's symptoms should be given, and the family should be helped to understand the child's underlying distress, but not accept this as an excuse for irresponsible behavior.

Some broad goals for therapy include the following (International Society for the Study of Dissociation 2004):

- Gradually helping the child achieve a sense of cohesion about his or her affects, cognitions, and associated behavior

- Enhancing motivation for growth and future success
- Promoting the child's self-acceptance of behavior and self-knowledge about feelings viewed as unacceptable.
- Helping the child to resolve conflicting feelings, wishes, loyalties, identifications, or contrasting expectations, which may result from existing family dysfunction.
- Desensitizing traumatic memories and correcting learned attitudes towards life resulting from traumatic events.
- Promoting autonomy and the child's ability to independently regulate and express affects using non-injurious mechanisms.
- Promoting healthy attachments and relationships through direct expression of feelings.

In addition to therapy, adjunctive therapeutic approaches may be employed, including the following (International Society for the Study of Dissociation 2004):

- *Family therapy*. These may include guidance on appropriate parenting strategies.
- *Pharmacotherapy*. There are no existing controlled studies evaluating the use of medications for children or adolescents with dissociative disorders. However, medications could be used to treat comorbid conditions such as depression, OCD, or post-traumatic stress disorder.
- *Group therapy*. This may be utilized for psychoeducational therapy, and may promote positive peer interaction.
- *Inpatient treatment*. This may be necessary when a child or adolescent is engaged in dangerous, self-injurious, or destructive behavior that cannot be managed in the community environment, or where the child is at imminent risk of harm and in need of a safe environment for complex assessment.
- *Educational interventions*. These may be required if the child's disruptive behavior, mood instability, and poor attention has interfered with academic function. Efforts should be made to discourage special attention from other students in the school environment.

REFERENCES

Adinkrah, M 2011, Epidemiologic characteristics of suicidal behavior in contemporary Ghana. *Crisis,* 32, 31–36.

Afifi, ZE, El-Lawindi, MI, Ahmed, SA and Basily, WW 2003, Adolescent abuse in a community sample in BeniSuef, Egypt: Prevalence and risk factors. *East Mediterr Health J,* 9, 1003–1018.

American Psychiatric Association 2013, *Diagnostic and Statistical Manual of Mental Disorders*, DSM-5, 5th Ed. Washington, DC: American Psychiatric Publishing.

Brown, DW, Riley, L, Butchart, A, Meddings, DR, Kann, L and Harvey, AP 2009, Exposure to physical and sexual violence and adverse health behaviours in African children: Results from the Global School-based Student Health Survey. *Bull World Health Organ,* 87, 447–455.

Burrows, S and Laflamme, L 2008, Suicide among urban South African adolescents. *Int J Adolesc Med Health,* 20, 519–528.

Cagiada, S, Candido, L and Pennati, A 1997, Successful integrated hypnotic and psychopharmacological treatment of war-related post-traumatic psychological and somatoform dissociative disorder of two years duration (psychogenic coma). *Dissociation,* 10, 182–189.

Department for International Development 2006, Annual Report.

Ghazinour, M, Emami, H, Richter, J, Abdollahi, M and Pazhumand, A 2009, Age and gender differences in the use of various poisoning methods for deliberate parasuicide cases admitted to loghman hospital in Tehran (2000–2004). *Suicide Life Threat Behav,* 39, 231–239.

Groohi, B, Rossignol, AM, Barrero, SP and Alaghehbandan, R 2006, Suicidal behavior by burns among adolescents in Kurdistan, Iran: A social tragedy. *Crisis,* 27, 16–21.

International Society for the Study of Dissociation 2004, Guidelines for the evaluation and treatment of dissociative symptoms in children and adolescents: International Society for the Study of Dissociation. *J Trauma Dissociation* [Internet], [cited 2016 Mar 25], 5(3), 119–50. Available at http://www.tandfonline.com/doi/abs/10.1300/J229v05n03_09

Laor, N, Wolmer, L, Kora, M, Yucel, D, Spirman, S and Yazgan, Y 2002, Post-traumatic, dissociative and grief symptoms in Turkish children exposed to the 1999 earthquakes. *J Nerv Ment Dis,* 190, 824–832.

Malemo Kalisya, L, Lussy Justin, P, Kimona, C, Nyavandu, K, Mukekulu Eugenie, K, Jonathan, KM, Claude, KM and Hawkes, M 2011, Sexual violence toward children and youth in war-torn eastern, Democratic Republic of Congo. *PLoS One,* 6, e15911.

Marder, SR, Sorsaburu, S, Dunayevich, E, Karagianis, JL, Dawe, IC, Falk, DM, Dellva, MA, Carlson, JL, Cavazzoni, PA and Baker, RW 2010, Case reports of post-marketing adverse event experiences with olanzapine intramuscular treatment in patients with agitation. *J Clin Psychiatry,* 71, 433–441.

Martin, A, Volmar, FR and Lewis, M (eds) 2007, *Lewis' child and adolescent psychiatry: A comprehensive textbook.* 4th ed. Philadelphia: Lippincott Williams and Wilkins.

Muula, AS, Kazembe, LN, Rudatsikira, E and Siziya, S 2007, Suicidal ideation and associated factors among in-school adolescents in Zambia. *Tanzan Health Res Bull,* 9, 202–206.

Nordstrom, K and Allen, MH 2007, Managing the acutely agitated and psychotic patient. *CNS Spectr,* 12 (10 Suppl 17), 5–11.

Oladokun, R, Brown, BJ, Osinusi, K, Akingbola, TS, Ajayi, SO and Omigbodun, OO 2008, A case of human bite by an 11 year old HIV positive girl in a Paediatric ward. *Afr J Med Med Sci,* 37, 81–85.

Omigbodun, O 2001, Sexual abuse among Nigerian youth: The remedy. Lecture delivered at the annual symposium of The Action Group on Adolescent Health (AGAH), University of Ibadan.

Omigbodun, O 2004, Psychosocial issues in a child and adolescent psychiatric clinic population in Nigeria. *Soc Psychiatry Psychiatr Epidemiol,* 39, 667–672.

Omigbodun, O, Dogra, N, Esan, O and Adedokun, B 2008, Prevalence and correlates of suicidal behaviour among adolescents in southwest Nigeria. *Int J Soc Psychiatry,* 54, 34–46.

Omigbodun, O and Olatawura, MO 2008, Child rearing practices in Nigeria: Implications for mental health. *Nigerian Journal of Psychiatry,* 6, 10–15.

Rudatsikira, E, Muula, AS, Siziya, S and Twa-Twa, J 2007, Suicidal ideation and associated factors among school-going adolescents in rural Uganda. *BMC Psychiatry,* 7, 67.

Schaffer, D, Gould, M and Hicks, R 2007, Teen suicide fact sheet. New York: Department of Child Psychiatry, New York State Psychiatric Institute, Columbia College of Physicians and Surgeons.

Scivoletto, S, Boarati, MA and Turkiewicz, G 2010, Psychiatric emergencies in childhood and adolescence. *Rev Bras Psiquiatr,* 32 (Suppl 2), 112–120.

Shipman, K and Taussig, H 2009, Mental health treatment of child abuse and neglect: The promise of evidence-based practice. *Pediatr Clin North Am,* 56, 417–428.

Smith, HA, Fuchs, DC, Pandharipande, PP, Barr, FE and Ely, EW 2009, Delirium: An emerging frontier in the management of critically ill children. *Crit Care Clin,* 25, 593–614.

Sorrentino, A 2004, Chemical restraints for the agitated, violent, or psychotic pediatric patient in the emergency department: Controversies and recommendations. *Curr Opin Pediatr,* 16, 201–205.

Wang, G, Fang, Y, Jiang, L, Zhou, G, Yuan, S, Wang, X and Sum, P 2015, [Relationship between cyberbullying and the suicide related psychological behavior among middle and high school students in Anhui Province]. *Wei Sheng Yan Jiu,* 44, 896–903.

Xing, XY, Tao, FB, Wan, YH, Xing, C, Qi, XY, Hao, JH, Su, PY, Pan, HF and Huang, L 2010, Family factors associated with suicide attempts among Chinese adolescent students: A national cross-sectional survey. *J Adolesc Health,* 46, 592–599.

Xing, Y, Qiao, Y, Duan, J and Bai, C 2015, [Prevalence of deliberate self-harm and its relation with suicidal behaviors among students in middle schools in Beijing]. *Zhonghua Liu Xing Bing Xue Za Zhi Zhonghua Liuxingbingxue Zazhi,* 36, 921–924.

Yéo-Tenena, YJ, Yao, YP, Bakayoko, AS, N'dja, GR, Kouamé, LM, Soro, SJ and Delafosse, RC 2010, Descriptive study of suicidal adolescents conducted in Abidjan. *Encephale,* 36 (Suppl 2), D41–D47.

11 Sexual Emergencies: A Psychiatrist's Perspective

T.S. Sathyanarayana Rao, Gurvinder Kalra

INTRODUCTION

Sexual health forms an important component of the overall health of an individual in addition to physical and mental health. Any problem or dysfunction in this area affects the individual's quality of life. Various specialists encounter patients with sexual problems that are present in an insidious form; however, to everyone's surprise, patients sometimes visit the emergency room (ER). Although psychiatrists may not have to be in the forefront in dealing with sexual emergencies, they sometimes have to work as part of a multidisciplinary team to deal with the after-effects of such emergencies in the ER.

Sexual emergencies can be classified into those that are real and affect the sexual organs and erogenous zones per se, and those that are perceived by patients as affecting their sexual organs or functioning, and hence, may not involve the sexual organs in its truest sense (Table 11.1). In a real sexual emergency, a psychiatrist may form part of a multidisciplinary team and play a crucial role in helping the patient. In a perceived sexual emergency, there are chances that the patient will consult a psychiatrist before consulting any other medical professional.

REAL SEXUAL EMERGENCIES

Men

Paraphimosis

Also known as capistration, paraphimosis is a urologic emergency and refers to the entrapment of a retracted foreskin behind the coronal sulcus. It usually occurs among uncircumcised or partially circumcised men. It may occur during coitus or when the individual retracts the foreskin and forgets to pull it back. Paraphimosis may be precipitated by penile piercing (Verma 2005; Raman, Kate and Ananthakrishnan 2008; Koenig and Carnes 1999). With time, the venous and lymphatic flow to the glans gets impaired, leading to engorgement and swelling of the glans. This compromises the arterial supply. If it is not treated in time, it may result in penile infarction, necrosis, gangrene, and eventually, auto-amputation (Raman, Kate and Ananthakrishnan 2008).

In the ER: Prompt attention and treatment usually lead to a favorable outcome.

TABLE 11.1

Classification of Sexual Emergencies

REAL		
Men	**Women**	**Gender-variant individuals**
Paraphimosis Priapism Penile fractures and other penile injuries Penile foreign bodies Acute reactions to sexual dysfunctions	Vaginal foreign bodies Vaginismus Vulvodynia	Acute emergencies in transsexuals during post-castration period
MISCELLANEOUS	Auto-asphyxiation Sexual assault Rectal foreign bodies	
PERCEIVED	Nuptial night anxiety Koro	

One should take a detailed history focusing on any instrumentation, circumcision, past history of paraphimosis, and sexually transmitted diseases. This should be followed by local examination to check for penile viability (Berk and Lee 2004). Although a urologic emergency, non-surgical methods can be used to reduce edema. These include squeezing the glans; injecting hyaluronidase; applying circumferential, compressive dressing, ice, or granulated sugar on the edematous prepuce and covering it with a condom; the "puncture" technique and direct blood aspiration (Berk and Lee 2004; Litzky 1997; Cahill and Rane 1999; Finkelstein 1994; Olson 1998; Choe 2000).

A psychiatrist's input may be required in the case of paraphimosis, such as when delayed help-seeking leads to complications such as loss of the penis. In such a case, it is important to assess the patient for underlying depressive features and other emotional turmoil, and help him deal with the feelings associated with a perceived loss of manhood or masculinity. Some patients may also need to be advised about the need for circumcision. It may be important to assess the patient for clinical syndrome of depression and treat it accordingly.

Priapism

Priapism refers to a persistent and painful penile erection not associated with sexual stimulation and unrelieved by ejaculation. It can be classified into three main types: Veno-occlusive (ischemic, low-flow resulting from failure of drainage of blood from erectile bodies due to prolonged blockage of draining veins), arterial (non-ischemic, high-flow due to unregulated flowing in of arterial blood into the erectile bodies secondary to a fistula between arteries and these bodies), and recurrent or stuttering priapism (Penaskovic, Haq and Raza 2010; Pryor *et al.* 2004). The first may be caused by prolonged relaxation of erectile smooth muscle due to drugs (penile injections, antidepressants, and antipsychotics) or due to sludging of blood in various blood disorders, such as sickle cell anemia and multiple myeloma (Thompson, Ware and Blashfield 1990; Morrison and Burnett 2011). Arterial priapism is usually the result of perineal or penile trauma, such as that seen in bicycle injuries or direct traumas.

In the ER: Acute treatment should be instituted to avoid the development of cavernosal fibrosis and permanent erectile dysfunction (Ashindoitiang 2010). Patients usually need to undergo drainage of blood from the penis (corporeal aspiration), and phenylephrine injection is usually required to facilitate smooth muscle contraction and detumescence (Pryor *et al.* 2004).

A psychiatrist may come across priapism in patients on various psychotropic drugs (Compton and Miller 2001). It is important for the psychiatrist to educate the patient on various side-effects of psychotropics including priapism, and to tell the patient to report urgently in case of persistent erection lasting for more than four hours (Pryor *et al.* 2004). Psychiatrists should recognize this complication and stop the offending drug immediately. There are case reports of priapism caused by risperidone, olanzapine, and quetiapine (Penaskovic, Haq and Raza 2010). Some patients report being stabilized on loxapine and standing pseudoephedrine to prevent any further priapistic episodes. Intracavernosal injection of vasoactive drugs (ICIVAD), such as papaverine and phentolamine, is also known to cause priapism. Detumescence is necessary and every practising doctor should be aware of this (Table 11.2). In fact, it is suggested that no clinician should undertake ICIVAD therapy unless they are willing and able to treat priapism. If priapism is not treated immediately, it can damage the patient's erectile capability permanently. The other acute complications of ICIVAD include ecchymoses, nodules, hematoma, and urethral bleeding (if wrongly injected into the spongiosums of the urethra). Long-term use of ICIVAD may lead to cavernosal fibrosis (Kulkarni 1998).

Penile Fracture

This is an uncommon condition which occurs when the erect penis bends abruptly and suddenly. The classic scenario in which it can occur is when a couple is having sexual intercourse in the passive partner-on-top position, the penis accidentally comes out of the penetrated area and the passive partner exerts the body weight downwards onto the penis. It may also occur during aggressive masturbation, when one rolls over onto

TABLE 11.2

Procedure for Detumescence in Priapism

Reassure the patient. Insert a 20-gauge scalp vein needle into one of the corpus cavernosa in the distal penile shaft and allow the blood to drain out into a sterile tray. Initially the blood may be dark red. After drainage of 50–300 mL, which should be done slowly over 15–90 minutes, the blood will turn bright red. Around this time, inject 0.02 mg of adrenaline (prepared by diluting 1 mg of adrenaline in 20 mL of saline; thus 1 mL=0.05 mg adrenaline) and clamp the scalp vein needle. Observe for 5 minutes. Watch for hypertension and arrhythmias. In elderly individuals, cardiac monitoring may be necessary. If the penis remains detumesced, then remove the needle and compress the penis for 5 minutes.

If the erection does not subside, repeat the procedure for draining blood for 15 minutes. This should be followed by another injection of adrenaline.

an erect penis during sleep, or due to a direct blow on the erect penis. Fibrosclerosis of the tunica albuginea and chronic urethritis predispose a person to penile fractures. The application of a force such as those described above produces a tear in the tunica albuginea, resulting in a sudden loss of erection (which, if absent, rules out a penile fracture). The other clinical features include sudden penile pain, penile bruising, bleeding, swelling, deviation and voiding difficulties, and blood in the urine (Eke 2002).

In the ER: Penile fracture is often described as a "first look diagnosis". It is essential to first take a thorough history focusing on the mode of injury. The patient is then asked to void. If he experiences any pain in the process, it points to a urethral tear (Martinez Portillo *et al.* 2003). An urgent urologic consultation is required to deal with this emergency. Surgery involves drainage of the hematoma and repair of the tear(s) in the tunica. Immediate surgical repair gives excellent results as compared to conservative treatment (Mansi *et al.* 1993). Sexual relations are to be avoided for around 4–6 weeks after the injury and repair. Failure to repair the tunical rupture is associated with the development of delayed penile curvature and possibly erectile dysfunction.

A psychiatrist may be asked to help the patient deal with the after-effects of the injury, which may include penile plaque or the formation of a fibrotic nodule, resulting in angulation, coital difficulty, urethral fistula, and erectile dysfunction, all of which may lead to relationship difficulties. Erectile dysfunction resulting from penile fractures responds to phosphodiesterase type 5 (PDE5) inhibitors or pharmacologically induced penile erection (PIPE) therapy (Eke 2002; Zargooshi 2009).

A similar, though rare, form of penile amputation may occur among psychiatric patients going through an acute exacerbation of psychotic episodes. There have also been cases of penile amputation by spouses, such as the case of Lorena Bobbit (Curtin 1994). If the patient's history suggests the presence of a psychiatric condition, management involves stabilization of the acute psychotic episode, followed by maintenance psychiatric treatment and prevention of further episodes of mutilation of other body parts. After resolution of the acute psychotic episode, the patient may express a desire for penile preservation.

Other Penile Injuries

Other penile injuries, such as laceration of the foreskin and tear of the frenulum, are uncommon (McCann 2005). At times, the tip of foreskin or scrotal skin gets entrapped in the teeth of the zipper of trousers, giving rise to a painful "zipper injury". This occurs more commonly among uncircumcised children than adults and is easy to manage surgically, by cutting the median bar of the zipper (McCann 2005; Strait 1999).

Penile Foreign Bodies

Adults may apply foreign bodies on the penis for sexual gratification and children may do so during play (Pastor Navarro *et al.* 2009). Engorgement of the penis by encircling objects such as rings (metallic or non-metallic) is an acute emergency and may lead to penile gangrene, if not treated in time (Bhat *et al.* 1991; Nuhu *et al.* 2009; Singh, Joshi and Jaura 2010).

In the ER: Foreign bodies that result in engorgement of the penis present a challenge to urologists. The treatment of the patient in the ER consists of urgent decompression of the constricted penis to facilitate free flow of blood and micturition (Perabo *et al.* 2002). A psychiatrist may have to evaluate the patient and help him deal with any events that follow the accident.

Acute Reactions in Sexual Dysfunction

Sexual dysfunctions are usually chronic, with the dysfunction developing gradually over months or even years. Psychological reactions that occur in response to these dysfunctions may develop gradually over time or in some cases, they may be acute, developing immediately after the realization of the loss of one's sexual functioning. The reactions could include shock, grief, anger, anxiety, hopelessness, sadness, and depression. A psychiatrist should do a comprehensive assessment of the patient and manage issues accordingly.

Women

Vaginal Foreign Bodies

It is most commonly children who are found to have vaginal foreign bodies (VFBs). Various types of VFBs have been reported (Meniru, Moore and Thomlinson 1996; Carey, Healy and Elder 2010). The foreign bodies may have been inserted into the vagina by the person herself for sexual gratification or they may have been inserted as part of a sexual assault (Carey, Healy and Elder 2010; Anderson and Anderson 1993). The presence of foreign bodies in the vagina can give rise to different types of fistulas, such as vesicovaginal, urethrovaginal, and rectovaginal (Carey, Healy and Elder 2010; Anderson and Anderson 1993; Hanai *et al.* 2000; Kobayashi *et al.* 2010).

In the ER: The patient may present with a history of frank vaginal bleeding and blood-stained or foul-smelling vaginal discharge. Smaller bodies might go unnoticed and remain asymptomatic for long periods of time. Definitive treatment consists of removing the VFB and treating any associated infection (Stricker, Navratil and Sennhauser 2004). Associated complications may have to be managed before the patient is fit for discharge from the medical facility.

A psychiatrist may have an important role to play if there is a history of sexual assault. This has been discussed in the section on sexual assault. The possibility of sexual abuse should always be kept in mind while evaluating girls or women with VFBs. Such evaluations may call for the skills of a psychiatrist or other mental health professionals (Herman-Giddens 1994; Sturgiss, Tyson and Parekh 2010).

Vaginismus

Vaginismus is an involuntary spasm of the muscles surrounding the vagina that makes intercourse painful and almost impossible. This condition is usually chronic. Most couples see a doctor late in their relationship and that, too, because they suspect infertility. However, some couples may present acutely, with the woman suffering from severe anxiety. Vaginismus is associated with several emotional difficulties, including low self-esteem, relationship issues, and depression with these being seen in either of the partners. It is crucial to address these issues, in addition to working on the patient's fears regarding vaginal penetration. Teaching the patient about vaginal exploration through touch, desensitization with vaginal dilators, sensate focus exercises, etc. can help to reduce the severity of vaginismus. Also, teaching the patient relaxation techniques and helping her deal with the accompanying emotional issues may go a long way in treating such cases.

Vulvodynia (or Burning Vagina Syndrome)

This is a syndrome of unexplained vulvar pain that is frequently associated with physical disabilities, limitation of daily activities, sexual dysfunction, and psychological issues (Friedrich 1987). Although it starts off as an acute problem, it may soon become chronic, lasting for months to years. According to patients, the pain is of a burning nature (McKay 1989). In the absence of any physical or laboratory findings, cases of vulvodynia may be referred to a psychiatrist (Ashman and Ott 1989). Treatment with tricyclic medications has proved successful in some patients.

Gender-variant Individuals

The transsexuals in India, called *hijras*, castrate or emasculate themselves in a ritual called *nirvan* (Kalra 2012). This ritual is usually, though not always, performed by traditional *dais* in the *hijra* clans. It is performed with the consent of the individual and usually under the influence of intoxicating substances. There are chances of some people suffering severe bleeding that may be life-threatening. Some individuals bleed to death due to untimely help, while very few reach the emergency department (ED) in need of urgent surgical intervention (Patwardhan *et al.* 2007).

A psychiatrist may have to help the patient deal with the emotions that could surface after initial stabilization. The emotions may range from guilt for having a failed nirvan (that may have psycho-socio-cultural significance for these individuals) to anger.

MISCELLANEOUS

Sexual Assault

The rate of sexual assault is increasing and such assaults can involve both women and men, though the latter are not very forthcoming about reporting them (Merchant *et al.* 2001). Anecdotal evidence also points to cases of sexual assault on transsexual and other gender-variant individuals. The use of force and weapons is common in such cases (Riggs *et al.* 2000). The presence of genital trauma is an important indicator of sexual abuse, although its absence does not rule out the same and many individuals may not have visible genital (or anal) injuries (Riggs *et al.* 2000; Palmer *et al.* 2004; Berkoff *et al.* 2008; Hilden, Schei and Sidenius 2005). There may be evidence of anal injuries and general body trauma. Genital injuries have been found to be present more commonly among younger victims and post-menopausal women than among individuals belonging to other age groups (Poulos and Sheridan 2008).

In the ER: It is important to perform a full genital examination and examine the whole body to look for injuries such as tears, abrasions, and bruises. However, the victim's informed consent must be taken before the examination. It is of vital importance to take a detailed history during such emergencies, but the clinician must do this in a sensitive manner to avoid making the victim feel ridiculed and humiliated. The clinician should be aware that any attempt at genital examination may trigger flashbacks of the sexual assault. Once the history and findings of the full examination have been documented in detail, the injuries must be given surgical attention. It is also crucial to test the patient for evidence of any sexually transmitted disease because of the high prevalence of such infections among victims of sexual assault (Siegel *et al.* 1995).

A psychiatrist plays a central role in cases of sexual assault by helping the victim deal with feelings of shock, anger, or denial in the acute stage immediately after the assault. Care must be taken to provide all help in a non-judgmental environment and to keep one's own emotions out of the picture. It is important to allow victims to ventilate their feelings, and this process can be facilitated by a psychiatrist or any other mental health professional. It is also crucial to restore a sense of psychological safety as victims of sexual assault are likely to feel that they are in danger and at risk of further assault. Victims may develop post-traumatic psychological stress syndrome as a result of the attack, and if this is not managed properly, it could give rise to both short- and long-term dysfunctional elements. Victims may require help to deal with feelings of self-blame and may need to be reassured that they are not to be blamed at all for the assault. Psychiatrists should lend their services to multidisciplinary teams dealing with cases of sexual assault, and should help develop psychological and social supportive services for such victims. Such teams may comprise medical, surgical, forensic, and social workers, among others. Providing psychological support, together with psychoeducation on the common reactions to such catastrophic events, may help reduce the victim's anxiety, guilt, and anger. The psychiatrist could also help and encourage the victim to take action on what has happened.

Rectal Foreign Bodies

It is not uncommon for patients to present to the ED with rectal foreign bodies. The nature of the rectal foreign body is said to be limited only by the imagination of the patient concerned (Manimaran, Shorafa and Eccersley 2009; Koornstra and Weersma 2008; Clarke *et al.* 2005; Wigle 1988). A person may insert a foreign body into the rectum to stimulate himself/herself sexually, may slip it in accidentally, or may even do so deliberately with the intention of concealing some substance (Clarke *et al.* 2005; Wigle 1988; Griffin and McGwin 2009; Yacobi, Tsivian and Sidi 2007). Patients may present with abdominal pain, pelvic, or anal discomfort and constipation. The presence of foreign bodies in the rectum can lead to various types of colorectal traumatic injuries, including rectal perforations and sphincter injuries; hence, it should be considered a serious condition and treated on an emergency basis (Ruiz *et al.* 2001; Rodriguez–Hermosa *et al.* 2007).

In the ER: A detailed clinical history, a physical examination, and a few diagnostic tests are essential for the diagnosis and management of lesions caused by rectal foreign bodies (Ruiz *et al.* 2001). The foreign bodies can be removed trans-anally with laparoscopic assistance or through the use of surgical approaches (Kantarian *et al.* 1987; Berghoff and Franklin 2005).

The psychiatrist needs to rule out any psychiatric illness in such cases, as according to some studies, rectal foreign bodies are commonly found among mentally ill patients, including those who use drugs and alcohol (Rodriguez–Hermosa *et al.* 2007). It is also essential to explore the possibility of sexual assault, especially in the case of mentally retarded children with rectal foreign bodies.

PERCEIVED SEXUAL PROBLEMS

Nuptial Night Anxiety (or Wedding Night Anxiety)

Sexual intercourse on the wedding night, an event much celebrated in many cultures, sometimes gives rise to significant levels of anxiety in both or either of the partners. Such anxiety commonly affects sexually inexperienced individuals who are worried about their performance and have high expectations from their first sexual encounter. In an attempt to prove his masculinity, the bridegroom may start focusing on getting an erection, which at times leads to failure to perform. Men usually suffer from premature ejaculation on such occasions. On the other hand, the bride may become overtly anxious about the outcomes of the first intercourse, especially the pain or bleeding that may occur as a result of the rupture of the hymen.

A psychiatrist can play an important role in dealing with distressed bridegrooms who present in the ER, seeking help. The psychiatrist can definitely bring down the bridegroom's anxiety level by helping him to relax and correct any misconceptions and preconceived notions. Learning about and understanding his expectations and teaching him about different phases of sexual intercourse may help in due course of time. The psychiatrist has to be aware of the possibility of stress of marriage triggering off any psychiatric disorder, e.g. acute nuptial psychosis (Mechri *et al.* 2000).

Koro

Patients with koro, which has been described as a culture-bound syndrome, experience sudden and intense anxiety due to the fear that the penis or even the entire male genitalia (vulva and nipples or breast in females) will recede into the body and possibly cause death. Koro may either be the primary disorder or secondary to other psychiatric disorders (schizophrenia, anxiety disorder, depression), diseases of the central nervous system (epilepsy, brain tumors), or withdrawal from drugs. Although the acute type of koro is more common, a less common chronic form has also been reported (Westermeyer 1989; Bernstein and Gaw 1990; Earleywine 2001; Kar 2005).

When a patient with koro visits the ER, one should rule out any other psychopathology or organic cause. While psychoeducation helps to relieve these symptoms in some cases, medications are required in other cases to reduce anxiety or take care of other psychiatric symptoms associated with the condition (Dutta 1983).

Other rare sexual emergencies that a psychiatrist may come across include cases of homosexual panic, which are more of historical importance nowadays, and even cases of gay individuals who are in a crisis about coming out before their family members.

CONCLUSION

While sexual emergencies constitute only a small percentage of the emergencies in any casualty department, these are the emergencies that may need a bit of extra attention from medical multidisciplinary teams. An extra effort is required to obtain a history of injury in such cases since the patient may act secretive. Although the primary aim would be to stabilize the patient, a psychiatrist may be called in at different points in time, either to obtain more details of the history or to help the patient ventilate. A psychiatrist thus needs to be prepared to deal with such patients rather than be clueless when faced with such cases in the ER.

REFERENCES

Anderson, PG and Anderson, M 1993, An unusual cause of rectovaginal fistula. *Aust NZ J Surg,* 63, 148–149.

Ashindoitiang, JA 2010, Management of priapism: A case report. *Nig Q J Hosp Med,* 20, 101–103.

Ashman, RB and Ott, AK 1989, Autoimmunity as a factor in recurrent vaginal candidosis and the minor vestibular gland syndrome. *J Reprod Med,* 34, 264–266.

Berghoff, KR and Franklin, ME Jr 2005, Laparoscopic-assisted rectal foreign body removal: Report of a case. *Dis Colon Rectum,* 48, 1975–1977.

Berk, DR and Lee, R 2004, Paraphimosis in a middle-aged adult after intercourse. *Am Fam Physician,* 69, 807–808.

Berkoff, MC, Zolotor, AJ, Makoroff, KL, Thackeray, JD, Shapiro, RA and Runyan, DK 2008, Has this prepubertal girl been sexually abused? *JAMA,* 300, 2779–2792.

Bernstein, RL and Gaw, AC 1990, Koro: Proposed classification for DSM-IV. *Am J Psychiatry,* 147, 1670–1674.

Bhat, AL, Kumar, A, Mathur, SC and Gangwal, KC 1991, Penile strangulation. *Br J Urol,* 68, 618–621.

Cahill, D and Rane, A 1999, Reduction of paraphimosis with granulated sugar. *BJU Int,* 83, 362.

Carey, R, Healy, C and Elder, DE 2010, Foreign body sexual assault complicated by rectovaginal fistula. *J Forensic Leg Med,* 17, 161–163.

Choe, JM 2000, Paraphimosis: Current treatment options. *Am Fam Physician,* 62, 2623–2626.

Clarke, DL, Buccimazza, I, Anderson, FA and Thomson, SR 2005, Colorectal foreign bodies. *Colorectal Dis,* 7, 98–103.

Compton, MT and Miller, AH 2001, Priapism associated with conventional and atypical antipsychotic medications: A review. *J Clin Psychiatry,* 62, 362–366.

Curtin, LL 1994, Morals: From Bobbit to Kevorkian. *Nurs Manage,* 25, 42–43.

Dutta, D 1983, Koro epidemic in Assam. *Br J Psychiatry,* 143, 309–310.

Earleywine, M 2001, Cannabis-induced koro in Americans. *Addiction,* 96, 1663–1666.

Eke, N 2002, Fracture of the penis. *Br J Surg,* 89, 555–565.

Finkelstein, JA 1994, 'Puncture' technique for treating paraphimosis. *Pediatr Emerg Care,* 10, 127.

Friedrich, EG Jr 1987, Vulvar vestibulitis syndrome. *J Reprod Med,* 32, 110–114.

Griffin, R and McGwin, G Jr 2009, Sexual stimulation device-related injuries. *J Sex Marital Ther,* 35, 253–261.

Hanai, T, Miyatake, R, Kato, Y and Iguchi, M 2000, Vesicovaginal fistula due to a vaginal foreign body: A case report. *Hinyokika Kiyo,* 46, 141–143.

Herman-Giddens, ME 1994, Vaginal foreign bodies and child sexual abuse. *Arch Pediatr Adolesc Med,* 148, 195–200.

Hilden, M, Schei, B and Sidenius, K 2005, Genitoanal injury in adult female victims of sexual assault. *Forensic Sci Int,* 154, 200–205.

Kalra, G 2012, Hijras: The unique transgender culture of India. *Int J Cult Mental Health,* 5, 121–126.

Kantarian, JC, Riether, RD, Sheets, JA, Stasik, JJ, Rosen, L and Khubchandani, IT 1987, Endoscopic retrieval of foreign bodies from the rectum. *Dis Colon Rectum,* 30, 902–904.

Kar, N 2005, Chronic koro-like symptoms – two case reports. *BMC Psychiatry,* 5, 34.

Kobayashi, K, Otoshi, T, Madono, K, Momohara, C, Imamura, R, Takada, S, Matsumiya, K, Fujita, M and Fukumoto, R 2010, A case of urethrovaginal fistula caused by a foreign body in the vagina. *Hinyokika Kiyo,* 56, 389–391.

Koenig, LM and Carnes, M 1999, Body piercing medical concerns with cutting-edge fashion. *J Gen Intern Med,* 14, 379–385.

Koornstra, JJ and Weersma, RK 2008, Management of rectal foreign bodies: Description of a new technique and clinical practice guidelines. *World J Gastroenterol,* 14, 4403–4406.

Kulkarni, V 1998, The injection erection. In: Brahmbhatt, R (ed). *Therapy of common sexual problems: A handbook,* pp. 66–72. Mumbai: Family Planning Association of India.

Litzky, GM 1997, Reduction of paraphimosis with hyaluronidase. *Urology,* 50, 160.

Manimaran, N, Shorafa, M and Eccersley, J 2009, Blow as well as pull: An innovative technique for dealing with a rectal foreign body. *Colorectal Dis,* 11, 325–326.

Mansi, MK, Emran, M, el-Mahrouky, A and el-Mateet, MS 1993, Experience with penile fractures in Egypt: Long-term results of immediate surgical repair. *J Trauma,* 35, 67–70.

Martínez Portillo, FJ, Seif, C, Braun, PM, Spahn, M, Alken, P and Jünemann, KP 2003, Penile fractures: Controversy of surgical vs. conservative treatment. *Aktuelle Urol,* 34, 33–36.

McCann, PA 2005, Case report: A novel solution to penile zipper-injury – the needle holder. *Scientific World Journal,* 5, 298–299.

McKay, M 1989, Vulvodynia: A multifactorial clinical problem. *Arch Dermatol,* 125, 256–262.

Mechri, A, Gaha, L, Khammouma, S, Skhiri, T, Zaafrane, F and Bedoui, A 2000, Acute nuptial psychosis: Apropos of 16 cases. *Encephale,* 26, 87–90.

Meniru, GI, Moore, J and Thomlinson, J 1996, Aerosol cap and rectovaginal fistula: Unusual findings at routine cervical smear. *Int J Gynaecol Obstet,* 52, 179–180.

Merchant, RC, Lau, TC, Liu, T, Mayer, KH and Becker, BM 2009, Adult sexual assault evaluations at Rhode Island emergency departments, 1995–2001. *J Urban Health,* 86, 43–53.

Morrison, BF and Burnett, AL 2011, Priapism in hematological and coagulative disorders: An update. *Nat Rev Urol,* 8, 223–230.

Nuhu, A, Edino, ST, Agbese, GO and Kallamu, M 2009, Penile gangrene due to strangulation by a metallic nut: A case report. *West Afr J Med,* 28, 340–342.

Olson, C 1998, Emergency treatment of paraphimosis. *Can Fam Physician,* 44, 1253–1254.

Palmer, CM, McNulty, AM, D'Este, C and Donovan, B 2004, Genital injuries in women reporting sexual assault. *Sex Health,* 1, 55–59.

Pastor Navarro, H, Donáte Moreno, MJ, Carrión López, P, Segura Martín, P, Lorenzo Romero, J, Pastor Guzmán, JM, Payá Berbegal, J, Lujan Marco, S and Virseda Rodríguez, J 2009, Penile foreign bodies. *Arch Esp Urol,* 62, 501–507.

Patwardhan, S, Sawant, A, Nagabhushana, M, Varma, R and Ismail, M 2007, Chronic urinary retention in eunuchs. *Indian J Urol,* 23, 317–318.

Penaskovic, KM, Haq, F and Raza, S 2010, Priapism during treatment with olanzapine, quetiapine, and risperidone in a patient with schizophrenia: A case report. *Prim Care Companion J Clin Psychiatry,* 12, PCC.09100939.

Perabo, FG, Steiner, G, Albers, P and Müller, SC 2002, Treatment of penile strangulation caused by constricting devices. *Urology,* 59, 137.

Poulos, CA and Sheridan, DJ 2008, Genital injuries in postmenopausal women after sexual assault. *J Elder Abuse Negl,* 20, 323–335.

Pryor, J, Akkus, E, Alter, G, Jordan, G, Lebret, T, Levine, L, Mulhall, J, Perovic, S, Ralph, D and Stackl, W 2004, Priapism. *J Sex Med,* 1, 116–120.

Raman, SR, Kate, V and Ananthakrishnan, N 2008, Coital paraphimosis causing penile necrosis. *Emerg Med J,* 25, 454.

Riggs, N, Houry, D, Long, G, Markovchick, V and Feldhaus, KM 2000, Analysis of 1,076 cases of sexual assault. *Ann Emerg Med,* 35, 358–362.

Rodríguez-Hermosa, JI, Codina-Cazador, A, Ruiz, B, Sirvent, JM, Roig, J and Farrés, R 2007, Management of foreign bodies in the rectum. *Colorectal Dis,* 9, 543–548.

Ruiz del Castillo, J, Sellés Dechent, R, Millán Scheiding, M, Zumárraga Navas, P and Asencio Arana, F 2001, Colorectal trauma caused by foreign bodies introduced during sexual activity: Diagnosis and management. *Rev Esp Enferm Dig,* 93, 631–634.

Siegel, RM, Schubert, CJ, Myers, PA and Shapiro, RA 1995, The prevalence of sexually transmitted diseases in children and adolescents evaluated for sexual abuse in Cincinnati: Rationale for limited STD testing in prepubertal girls. *Pediatrics,* 96, 1090–1094.

Singh, I, Joshi, MK and Jaura, MS 2010, Strangulation of penis by a ball-bearing device. *J Sex Med,* 7, 3793–3797.

Strait, RT 1999, A novel method for removal of penile zipper entrapment. *Pediatr Emerg Care,* 15, 412–413.

Stricker, T, Navratil, F and Sennhauser, FH 2004, Vaginal foreign bodies. *J Paediatr Child Health,* 40, 205–207.

Sturgiss, EA, Tyson, A and Parekh, V 2010, Characteristics of sexual assaults in which adult victims report penetration by a foreign object. *J Forensic Leg Med,* 17, 140–142.

Thompson, JW Jr, Ware, MR and Blashfield, RK 1990, Psychotropic medication and priapism: A comprehensive review. *J Clin Psychiatry,* 51, 430–433.

Verma, S 2005, Coital penile trauma with severe paraphimosis. *J Eur Acad Dermatol Venereol,* 19, 134–135.

Westermeyer, J 1989, A case of koro in a refugee family: Association with depression and folie a deux. *J Clin Psychiatry,* 50, 181–183.

Wigle, RL 1988, Emergency department management of retained rectal foreign bodies. *Am J Emerg Med,* 6, 385–389.

Yacobi, Y, Tsivian, A and Sidi, AA 2007, Emergent and surgical interventions for injuries associated with eroticism: A review. *J Trauma,* 62, 1522–1530.

Zargooshi, J 2009, Sexual function and tunica albuginea wound healing following penile fracture: An 18-year follow-up of 352 patients from Kermanshah, Iran. *J Sex Med,* 6, 1141–1150.

12 Psychiatric Emergencies in Medical Conditions

Anju Kuruvilla, Anoop Raveendran, K.S. Jacob

Psychiatric emergencies, marked by severe disturbance of mood, thought, or behavior that require immediate attention, sometimes occur in non-psychiatric settings such as the general medical ward. No time should be lost in recognizing and evaluating these emergencies and managing them appropriately to prevent further complications. These complications could relate to the patient's disease state or it could be that the patient might pose a danger to himself and others.

Many medical conditions can give rise to psychiatric manifestations. The common psychiatric presentations seen in medical settings that require urgent intervention are agitation, violence, extreme distress, and suicidal behavior. These may be secondary to a variety of underlying conditions, including delirium, general medical conditions, diseases of the central nervous system, psychosis, and substance intoxication and withdrawal.

A thorough medical evaluation, including a detailed history, physical examination, and investigations are essential components of assessment. There are certain clinical features that are characteristic of psychiatric symptoms that occur secondary to medical conditions; these are listed in Box 12.1. Investigations in such cases should focus on the identification of organic and drug-induced psychiatric disorders as well as the physical consequences of the psychiatric disorder or substance abuse. While all tests may not be necessary in every case, appropriate investigations must be carried out depending on the clinical features (Box 12.2) (Khouzam, Tan and Gill 2007).

Many psychiatric symptoms that are secondary to medical illness may resolve with the treatment of the medical condition. Those who have a pre-existing or independent psychiatric disorder need simultaneous and ongoing treatment of both the medical and psychiatric conditions. Consultation with medical, neurological and other specialties helps to ensure appropriate management.

SOME COMMON GENERAL MEDICAL CONDITIONS THAT CAN GIVE RISE TO PSYCHIATRIC SYMPTOMS

Metabolic Disorders

- Hyponatremia: Irritability, depression, intense anxiety, psychosis, confusion

BOX 12.1 COMMON CHARACTERISTICS OF PSYCHIATRIC SYMPTOMS ACCOMPANYING MEDICAL CONDITIONS

- *Onset:* Sudden onset, late age of initial presentation
- *Past medical history:* Present
- *Past psychiatric history:* Absent
- *Symptom presentation:* Atypical presentation, disproportionate severity of behavioral disturbance compared with what is expected in a psychiatric condition
- *Mental state:* Memory dysfunction, disorientation, fluctuating level of consciousness
- *Symptom progression:* Temporal relationship between the onset, progression, exacerbation or remission of psychiatric symptoms, and the treatment of the medical condition; change in pattern of symptoms
- *Comorbidity:* Pre-existing systemic diseases; alcohol or substance intoxication/ withdrawal; use of prescription medications with psychiatric side-effects
- *Physical examination:* Presence of one or more abnormal vital signs or abnormal neurological findings
- *Treatment response:* Treatment resistance or unusual response to treatment

BOX 12.2 DIAGNOSTIC EVALUATION OF EMERGENCY PSYCHIATRIC PRESENTATIONS IN GENERAL MEDICAL SETTINGS

- Vital signs – pulse rate, blood pressure, respiratory rate, hydration, temperature
- Breath alcohol and blood alcohol levels
- Total and differential blood counts
- Hemoglobin
- Blood sugars
- Electrolytes
- Renal, liver, and thyroid function tests
- Blood urea nitrogen
- Vitamin B12 and folate levels
- Urine microscopy and drug screen
- Lumbar puncture and evaluation of the cerebrospinal fluid (CSF)
- Chest X-ray
- Electrocardiogram (ECG)
- Electroencephalogram (EEG)
- CT or MRI of the brain

- *Hypokalemia:* Apathy, weakness, confusion
- *Hepatic encephalopathy:* Delirium, abrupt behavioral changes, disinhibition, depression, hypomania, anxiety
- *Acute intermittent porphyria:* Psychosis
- *Wilson disease:* Personality changes, mood disturbances, depression, anxiety, phobias, poor memory

Degenerative/Demyelinating Disease

- *Parkinson disease:* Depression, anxiety, psychosis, cognitive impairment
- *Multiple sclerosis:* Memory loss, impairment in reasoning, planning, and organizational skills, dementia, personality changes, mood disorder, emotional dyscontrol
- *Creutzfeldt–Jakob disease:* Personality changes, hallucinations, confusion, disorientation, delirium, dementia

Head Trauma

- Inattention, poor concentration, impaired memory and judgment, depression, irritability, emotional outbursts, slowed thinking

Epilepsy

- Pseudoseizures, depression, anxiety, adjustment disorders, mania, psychosis, personality changes, cognitive impairment

Structural Disorders

- *Brain tumors:* Delirium
- *Frontal lobe tumors:* Cognitive impairment, personality change, motor and language dysfunction
- *Temporal lobe:* Memory and speech abnormalities, auditory hallucinations
- *Temporal, parietal and occipital lobe:* Visual hallucinations
- *Limbic and hypothalamic tumors:* Rage, mania, emotional lability, altered sexual behavior, delusions
- *Normal pressure hydrocephalus:* Cognitive impairment, depression

Toxins/Heavy Metals

- *Organophosphates:* Depression, impaired judgment and cognition, delirium, psychosis
- *Atropine:* Cognitive impairment, psychosis, delirium
- *Cyanide:* Anxiety, confusion
- *Mycotoxins:* Psychosis, anxiety, agitation

Infection/Sepsis

- *Neurosyphilis, Lyme disease:* Personality changes, disinhibition, impulsivity; irritability, delusions of grandeur, mania; decreased self-care, dementia
- *Meningitis:* Acute confusion, memory impairment, psychosis

- *Herpes simplex encephalitis:* Bizarre behavior, delirium, seizures, olfactory and gustatory hallucinations, personality changes, psychosis
- *Rabies encephalitis:* Hallucinations, overactivity, restlessness, agitation

Drug Abuse Toxicity or Withdrawal

- The clinical symptoms are related to the specific substance.
- *Alcohol:* Delirium, Wernicke encephalopathy (ophthalmoplegia, global confusional state, ataxia), Korsakoff syndrome (amnesia, confabulation), alcohol-induced mood or psychotic disorders

Medication

- Antihypertensives: Depression
- Oral contraceptives: Mood changes
- Steroids: Mood changes, psychosis
- Antituberculous drugs: Psychosis
- Anticholinergics: Delirium
- Antiparkinsonian agents: Depression, psychosis
- Zidovudine: Mania, anxiety, auditory hallucinations, confusion
- Cancer chemotherapy agents: Delirium, anxiety, depression, psychosis

Endocrinopathies

- *Pancreatic tumors:* Depression
- *Other pancreatic disorders*: Delirium
- *Hyperthyroidism:* Anxiety, agitated depression, mania, psychosis, delirium, confusion
- *Hypothyroidism:* Apathy, psychomotor retardation, depression, cognitive decline, mania, delirium, psychosis
- *Parathyroid disorders:* Delirium, sudden cognitive decline, depression, anxiety, psychosis, apathy
- *Cushing syndrome:* Depression, memory deficits, psychosis
- *Addison disease:* Irritability, apathy, fatigue, depression, psychosis, confusion
- *Pheochromocytoma:* Anxiety, sense of doom, delirium

Nutritional/Vitamin Deficiency

- *Thiamine:* Fatigue, depressed mood, confusion, Wernicke encephalopathy
- *Cobalamin:* Depression, fatigue, psychosis, progressive cognitive impairment
- *Folate:* Depression, cognitive impairment
- *Niacin:* Delirium, depression, mania, paranoid ideation
- *Pyridoxine:* Irritablity, nervousness, insomnia

Immunological/Inflammatory

- *Systemic lupus erythematosus:* Depression, emotional lability, delirium, psychosis

Vascular Disorders (Cardiac, Cardiopulmonary, Blood Vessels, Cerebrovascular, Embolism)

- Anxiety, panic, depression, insomnia, agitation, restlessness, violence, disorientation, confusion

MEDICATION MANAGEMENT OF EMERGENCY PSYCHIATRIC CONDITIONS IN GENERAL MEDICAL SETTINGS

In emergency situations, while the treatment of the underlying disorder is of key importance, it may be necessary to medicate the patient to calm him or her down prior to, and in order to, facilitate a detailed evaluation (Fig. 12.1).

Principles

- In the medically ill, medication should be started at lower doses and increased slowly.
- The lowest effective dose of medication should be used.
- The least number of medications should be used, and the need to use them must be reviewed every 24 hours, especially in those who are delirious.
- The patient should be monitored closely for side-effects to the prescribed medication, especially neurological, metabolic, and cardiac.
- The potential for drug interactions must be kept in mind as the patient is often on several other medications for different medical indications.
- In patients with renal impairment, one should avoid drugs that are nephrotoxic, those that are extensively renally cleared, as well as long-acting preparations.
- Whenever required, sedation should be incorporated into the core treatment by using antipsychotic or antidepressant medication that have sedative properties
- If benzodiazepines are used for symptomatic management, they must be carefully titrated and their use restricted to 4 weeks.
- Preferably, medication should be administered orally. However, parenteral preparations may be required in emergency situations as they have a faster onset of action; they may also be required in patients who may not be cooperative with or unable to take oral medication. Mouth dissolving preparations may be used if necessary.

Commonly Used Medication in Emergency Situations

Benzodiazepines

The benzodiazepine used most commonly in emergency situations is injectable or oral lorazepam, in a dose of 1–2 mg. It produces sedation and has a calming effect. Intramuscular administration is often necessary in an emergency when a very agitated patient is being uncooperative with oral treatment. The dose may be repeated to add up to a maximum of 8–10 mg a day. Lorazepam is fast-acting, easy to administer, and more reliably and consistently absorbed than other benzodiazepines when given intramuscularly. In agitated patients, it can be given singly, alternately with, or in combination with haloperidol. Some studies have indicated that the combination works

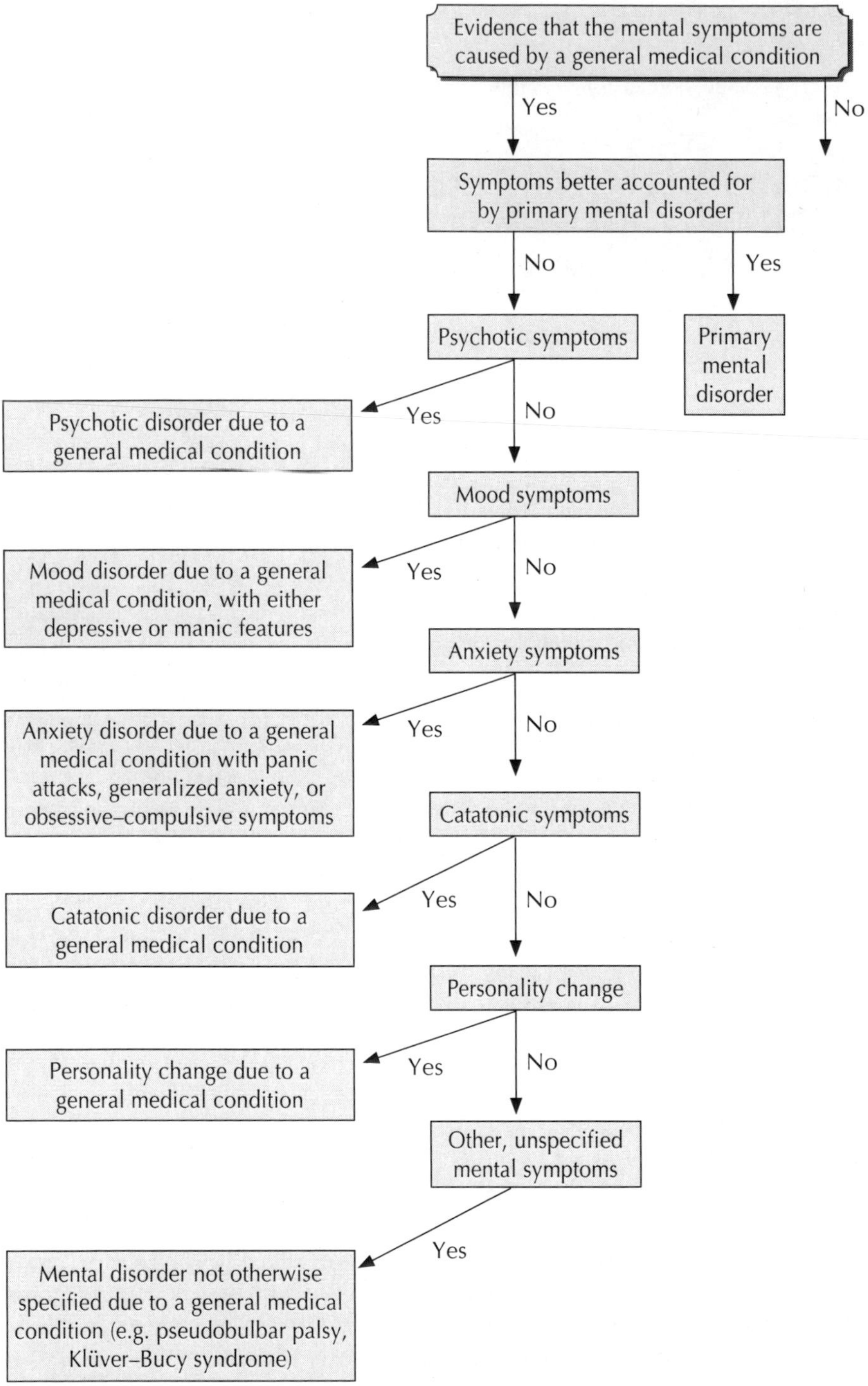

Figure 12.1 Algorithm for assessing and managing psychiatric illnesses due to a general medical condition

TABLE 12.1

Commonly Prescribed Benzodiazepines

Drug	Initial dose (mg)	Daily dose range (mg)
Alprazolam	0.25–0.5	1–6
Chlordiazepoxide	5–10	5–100
Clonazepam	0.25	0.5–6
Diazepam	2.5	5–40

more rapidly and may be more effective than either treatment alone, and is especially useful in patients who can tolerate only lower doses of antipsychotic medications or in whom anxiety or agitation is prominent (Battaglia *et al.* 1997; Bieniek *et al.* 1998).

Other benzodiazepines that are commonly prescribed are listed in Table 12.1. These are to be taken orally.

Common Emergency Indications

- Monotherapy with benzodiazepines is generally reserved for patients with delirium secondary to substance withdrawal and seizures
- Agitation, anxiety, depression
- Psychosis
- Situations in which antipsychotic medication is contraindicated, e.g. neuroleptic malignant syndrome

Precautions

- When used, benzodiazepines must be prescribed for short periods under supervision, and should be tapered and stopped within 3–4 weeks, as they are addictive.
- Benzodiazepines can cause respiratory depression, especially in the debilitated and those with respiratory ailments.
- Benzodiazepines are best avoided in older people.
- In delirious patients, other than those with delirium secondary to substance withdrawal and seizures, benzodiazepines can worsen confusion.

Antipsychotics

The most commonly used antipsychotic agent in emergency situations is haloperidol, considered a safe drug in medically ill patients. This high-potency typical antipsychotic is commonly administered intramuscularly in doses of 5–10 mg in emergency situations, when patients are acutely disturbed or refusing oral medication. While the dose may be repeated to add up to a maximum of 10–20 mg per day in the case of a patient with functional psychosis, lower doses must be used in patients with delirium (discussed below) and medical illnesses. Haloperidol injections may be combined with lorazepam or anticholinergic agents, such as benztropine and promethazine (25–50 mg). These drugs enhance the sedative effects of haloperidol, and the latter also reduce side-effects such as dystonia.

Olanzapine, an atypical antipsychotic, is now available for intramuscular administration. It can be administered at doses of 5–10 mg and repeated every 2 hours, the maximum dosage being 30 mg every 24 hours. However, for patients with dementia, the recommended dose is 2.5 mg. Oral administration of olanzapine is also useful as it produces sedation and reduces agitation (Breier *et al.* 2002).

Oral antipsychotic medications commonly used in this group of patients include haloperidol (2.5–5 mg), olanzapine (5–10 mg), quetiapine (25–100 mg) and risperidone (1–2 mg). The dose may be repeated every hour, if required. While chlorpromazine is an effective antipsychotic with sedative properties, the patient requires close monitoring because of the anticholinergic, sedative and hypotensive side-effects of the drug.

Common Emergency Indications

- Delirium
- Organic or functional psychosis
- Organic or functional mania
- Extreme agitation, anxiety or aggression

Precautions

- Patients who are medically ill may not be able to tolerate the doses usually prescribed to healthy patients with psychiatric symptoms and may be more susceptible to side-effects.
- Antipsychotic medication (especially the typical agents) produces acute extra-pyramidal side-effects, such as dystonia, akathisia, and drug-induced parkinsonism (tremor, rigidity, and bradykinesia). Tardive dyskinesia could occur with long-term use.
- The cardiac side-effects of antipsychotic medication that need to be closely monitored include alpha-1 adrenergic blockade (which occurs especially with the low-potency agents, such as chlorpromazine) and potential prolongation of the QTc interval (which is greater when the drug is used in combination with other medication with similar effects).
- Intramuscular administration of olanzapine may produce sedation and orthostatic hypotension.
- Anticholinergic drugs, used to reduce extrapyramidal side-effects, can worsen delirium.
- Patients with renal disease must be prescribed lower doses.

Antidepressants

Antidepressants are not usually prescribed for the immediate management of emergency presentations. If used in agitated or anxious patients, the choice of the antidepressant depends on factors such as comorbid medical illnesses, concurrent medication, potential drug interactions, and the side-effect profile of the antidepressant agent. The use of tricyclic antidepressants can result in postural hypotension, cardiac arrhythmias, and conduction disturbances, in addition to anticholinergic effects.

Mood Stabilizers

Mood stabilizers are commenced along with antipsychotics for their curative and prophylactic properties. The level of lithium, if prescribed, must be carefully monitored in view of its narrow therapeutic window. Its interactions with diuretics, angiotensin-converting enzyme (ACE) inhibitors and non-steroidal anti-inflammatory drugs (NSAIDs), as well as its effects on renal and thyroid functions, need to be kept in mind. The patient's liver function and blood counts need to be monitored carefully when sodium valproate and carbamazepine are used. Drug interactions are common with both these medicines, e.g. valproate displaces less protein-bound drugs, such as warfarin, leading to higher blood levels of those drugs.

Anticholinergic Medication

Anticholinergic medication is often used to reduce the extrapyramidal effects produced by antipsychotics. The commonly prescribed oral medications include trihexiphenidyl (2–8 mg/day) and benztropine (1–6 mg/day). Injectable benztropine (1–2 mg) and promethazine (25–50 mg) may be used intramuscularly (i.m.) or intravenously (i.v.) for immediate relief of acute dystonia. Promethazine may be used in combination with a haloperidol injection to enhance its sedative properties. Anticholinergic drugs can worsen confusion in patients with delirium and dementia. They can result in reduced gastrointestinal motility, urinary hesitancy, cardiac conduction problems, and drying of secretions. They should be used with caution in patients with glaucoma.

COMMON EMERGENCY PSYCHIATRIC PRESENTATIONS IN GENERAL MEDICAL SETTINGS

Agitation

Agitation is described as excessive verbal and/or motor behavior which can escalate to verbal or physical aggression (Box 12.3).

In a general medical setting, delirium is the commonest organic syndrome that results in agitation and must be ruled out before any other cause is assumed. Delirium itself may be the result of a myriad of medical conditions, or may be related to substance intoxication or withdrawal, or to medication. Delirium is characterized by the acute onset of an alteration in consciousness with a reduced ability to focus, sustain, or shift attention. This is accompanied by disorientation, language, and perceptual disturbances and memory deficits. The condition tends to fluctuate during the course of the day.

Dementia, more common in older people, is characterized by multiple cognitive dysfunctions, including a progressive deterioration in memory. It is associated with aphasia, apraxia, agnosia, and loss of executive function.

In the absence of alteration in consciousness and orientation, violence or agitation may indicate psychosis, mania, depression, anxiety, or an underlying personality disorder. Taking a thorough history and carrying out the relevant investigations can help to distinguish between organic conditions and purely functional ones.

Alcohol intoxication is characterized by disinhibition in normal social functioning. The person may be aggressive and lack coordination; speech may be loud, excessive,

BOX 12.3 DIFFERENTIAL DIAGNOSIS OF ACUTE AGITATION IN MEDICAL SETTINGS

- Delirium
- Dementia
- Substance use disorders
  - intoxication
  - withdrawal
- Psychosis
  - secondary to organic illness
  - functional
- Mania
  - secondary to organic illness
  - functional
- Depression-anxiety
  - secondary to organic illness
  - primary anxiety disorders
  - stress-related or adjustment difficulty
- Personality disorder
  - poor coping skills and impulse control
  - antisocial and borderline traits
- Medication-related
  - acute dystonic reaction
  - akathisia
  - neuroleptic malignant syndrome
  - anticholinergic delirium
  - theophylline related
- Medical and neurological disorders
  - brain injuries, brain tumors, metabolic disturbances, seizure disorder
- Pain
- Chaotic environment

and slurred; withdrawal is characterized by restlessness, tremors, sweating, anxiety, nausea, and vomiting; tachycardia and systolic hypertension may be evident. Seizures and delirium can also occur secondary to withdrawal.

Psychosis is characterized by delusions and hallucinations, along with disorganization in speech, thought, and behavior. Agitation is often secondary to paranoid delusions or hallucinations. Psychotic symptoms may occur secondary to organic pathology or may be purely functional in origin.

Patients with mania may be irritable or elated, expansive in mood, with pressured speech and hyperactivity which is goal-directed. Depressed individuals may report sadness, anxiety and feelings of guilt, worthlessness, hopelessness, and helplessness. Both these mood states may occur secondary to an organic etiology.

Intense anxiety, fear of impending doom, hyperventilation, and signs and symptoms of autonomic hyperactivity are observed in individuals having a panic attack. Occasionally, individuals who are in a state of acute stress secondary to emotional upheaval may present with agitation. Organic conditions may also give rise to manifestations of anxiety.

Clinical Assessment of Agitation

The patient's history must be taken and a physical examination, including neurological, as well as the mental state examination, need to be carried out. Their medical and psychiatric records, together with records of any operations, must be reviewed. The risk of violence needs to be assessed; a past history of violence and current delusions often predict future violent behavior. All medication being taken by the patient must be reviewed carefully and correlated with the behavioral changes. It is essential to assess the patient for the presence of delirium and cognitive impairment. One must check if there is a temporal relationship between the symptoms and a physical illness or substance abuse. The patient should be screened for major mental illnesses, such as psychosis, mood and anxiety disorders. Relevant investigations such as blood tests, neuroimaging, and an electroencephalogram may be required.

Medical Management of Agitation

- Observation and monitoring of the patient's general medical condition have to be stepped up. This includes frequent monitoring of the vital signs, fluid intake and output, and levels of oxygenation.
- Any underlying metabolic, toxic, infectious, or other non-psychiatric causes must be identified and treated. Vitamin supplements should be provided to patients with alcoholic delirium or those who are malnourished.
- *Sedation must be provided to the patient.* Lorazepam is a reasonable choice when treating an acute episode of agitation, especially when the etiology is not clear. Antipsychotic agents are the other group of medications commonly used.
- *The ideal treatment is parsimonious.* It should treat both the manifestations of agitation and the underlying illness. Examples are intramuscular haloperidol in schizophrenia and benzodiazepines in a panic attack.
- Intramuscular injection has a faster onset of action than oral or sublingual administration.
- Once the acute episode has been managed, strategies must be put in place to prevent subsequent episodes and manage the underlying clinical problem. The therapeutic approaches include the prescription of antipsychotic agents for psychosis, mood stabilizers for bipolar disorder, antidepressants and beta blockers for anxiety and depression, electroconvulsive therapy (ECT) for patients in whom other approaches have failed and psychological measures appropriate to the patient.
- The following are the principles of the management of medication in cases of delirium (Gleason 2003). The medication commonly used in delirium is listed in Table 12.2 (Taylor, Paton and Kerwin 2007).
  - Antipsychotics are the medication of choice.

TABLE 12.2

Medication Commonly Used in Delirium

Drug	Dose	Comments
Haloperidol	**Oral, 0.5–1 mg bd** Can be repeated every 4–6 hours, if required **Intramuscular, 0.5–1 mg** Can be repeated after 30–60 minutes, if required	Considered first-line agent Avoid in neuroleptic malignant syndrome, hepatic failure and anticholinergic toxicity Monitor for extrapyramidal symptoms, QTc interval
Quetiapine	**Oral, 12.5–25 mg bd** Can be increased every 1–2 days to 100 mg, if well tolerated	Monitor QTc interval Risperidone and olanzapine are considered to increase the risk of stroke among older patients with dementia
Risperidone	**Oral, 0.5 mg bd** Additional doses can be given every 4 hours, as needed	
Olanzapine	**Oral, 2.5–5 mg od**	
Lorazepam	**Oral/i.m., 0.5–1 mg** Every 2–4 hours, as needed	Used in delirium associated with alcohol/sedative hypnotic withdrawal, neuroleptic malignant syndrome Can cause respiratory depression, excessive sedation and paradoxical excitement

- Benzodiazepines should be reserved for delirium resulting from seizures or withdrawal from alcohol/sedative hypnotics, and can be used when unknown substances may have been ingested (Cook 2004).
- Antipsychotic drugs should be started at low doses, and should only be increased very gradually.
- Anticholinergic medication should be avoided as it can increase confusion and worsen memory impairment.
- The minimum number of medications should be used and the need for these must be reviewed every 24 hours.
- An attempt must be made to gradually discontinue medication 7–10 days after the symptoms resolve.

Non-pharmacological Management

Environmental: The patient should be provided with a calm environment in which there is adequate lighting. It must be ensured that the room does not have objects which could be used as weapons. The door should be kept open, and the patient and physician should be at an equal distance from the exit so that the physician has easy access to it in case the patient turns aggressive. The physician should stand at an angle and keep his hands visible.

Behavioral: The talking down approach may be used to de-escalate agitation. It is important to give the patient adequate space and to maintain a calm, relaxed manner while making normal eye contact. One should express genuine interest in the patient's problem and reassure them that they will come to no harm. The patient should be offered help, as well as choices, where possible, with both alternatives being safe ones. Offering choices allows the patient to participate in his own care and strengthens the therapeutic alliance. It is best to ask open-ended questions and communicate in clear, simple language. In cases of delirium, the patient should be reoriented to person, place, time, and circumstances. One should listen and avoid arguments. The consequences of inappropriate behavior should be mentioned without resorting to threats or anger. Relaxation techniques, such as deep breathing exercises, may be suggested.

Education: A therapeutic alliance needs to be established with the patient and the family, and it is important to educate them on the nature of the problem, its management, and the prognosis.

Some other conditions which can bring a patient to the medical emergency department are acute anxiety, suicidal behavior, and catatonia. These are dealt with in Chapters 1, 3, and 8.

Psychiatric Emergencies Among Patients with HIV

Among some patients with HIV, psychiatric disorders predate the HIV infection, while in others, they occur during the course of living with the disease and as a result of its psychosocial consequences. In yet other cases, the psychiatric disorder may be attributable to the direct neuropathic effects of the infection, or it may be secondary to opportunistic infections, secondary to the drugs that are used in treatment, or secondary to substance use disorders (Chandra, Desai and Ranjan 2005). A combination of the above factors may also give rise to the disorder. The psychiatric illness is often associated with poorer functioning and quality of life. Given the complex nature of the illness and its comorbidities, a variety of psychiatric emergencies can occur in patients with HIV infection. These include delirium, cognitive disorders, psychosis, mood and anxiety disorders, adjustment disorders, suicidality and substance intoxication or withdrawal (Bennett *et al.* 2009; McDaniel *et al.* 2010; Halstead *et al.* 1988; Harris *et al.* 1991).

GENERAL PRINCIPLES OF DRUG MANAGEMENT

- Symptomatic treatment of psychiatric symptoms is recommended.
- It is best to start at low doses and increase them cautiously as individuals with HIV are more susceptible to the side-effects of drugs and drug interactions.
- One should select the simplest dose regimen possible.

- The potential for drug interactions must be kept in mind as the patient is often on multiple other drugs for different medical indications.
- Benzodiazepines must be used with caution in view of potential drug interactions and the risk of misuse.
- *Antidepressants:* Selective serotonin reuptake inhibitors (SSRIs) or tricyclics may be used. It is advisable to use tricyclic agents cautiously in view of their potential side-effects.
- *Mood stabilizers:* Lithium is best avoided because of the relatively greater risk of toxicity and drug interactions. Carbamazepine tends to have interactions with antiretroviral agents and can cause agranulocytosis. Sodium valproate may be used cautiously. Liver function tests and the hemopoeitic system must be monitored carefully.
- The patient's medical status must be monitored carefully.

ADJUSTMENT DISORDERS

Acute anxiety, distress, agitation, and suicidal ideation may occur after the patient is informed of the diagnosis of HIV. They may also result from concerns related to the stigma associated with HIV, grief due to the prognosis and issues of loss. Benzodiazepines and antidepressants may be used.

HIV NEUROCOGNITIVE DISORDERS

Cognitive impairment can occur at any time in the course of the infection and can range from mild forgetfulness to severe dementia. While the symptoms commonly found among patients with HIV-associated dementia are memory impairment, psychomotor speed impairments, and movement disorders, the patient may also present with agitation, irritability, restlessness, anxiety, psychosis, or mood symptoms that require urgent intervention. The treatment includes symptomatic management with antipsychotics or antidepressants, as appropriate, in addition to highly active antiretroviral therapy (HAART) medication. The medical problems of the patient need to be identified and treated. The patient's safety should be ensured. The provision of support to the patient and his family is essential.

MOOD AND PSYCHOTIC SYMPTOMS

New onset of mood and psychotic syndromes may be seen in people with HIV, in the absence of medical or iatrogenic causes or concurrent substance abuse. In contrast to mania that occurs as part of a pre-existing bipolar disorder, the condition of these patients is often characterized by cognitive slowing and irritability rather than euphoria, and has a more severe and chronic course. In the early stages of the illness, the patient may be treated with traditional mood stabilizers and antipsychotics; however, in the later stages, patients are much more sensitive to the side-effects of drugs and will require smaller doses and careful titration. Electroconvulsive therapy may need to be considered for severe depression or mania, and antidepressants for depression.

TABLE 12.3

Neuropsychiatric Side-effects of Selected Medications Used for HIV Disease

Drug	Target illness	Side-effects
Acyclovir	Herpes encephalitis	Visual hallucinations, depersonalization, tearfulness, confusion, hyperesthesia, hyperacusis, thought insertion, insomnia
Amphotericin B	Cryptococcosis	Delirium, peripheral neuropathy, diplopia
β-lactam antibiotics	Infections	Confusion, paranoia, hallucinations, mania, coma
Cotrimoxazole	*Pneumocystis carinii* pneumonia	Depression, loss of appetite, insomnia, apathy
Cycloserine	Tuberculosis	Psychosis, somnolence, depression, confusion, tremors, vertigo, paresis, seizures, dysarthria
Didanosine	HIV	Nervousness, anxiety, confusion, seizures, insomnia, peripheral neuropathy
Efavirenz	HIV	Nightmares, depression, confusion
Foscarnet	Cytomegalovirus	Paresthesias, seizures, headache, irritability, hallucinations, confusion
Interferon-α	Kaposi sarcoma	Depression, weakness, headache, myalgias, confusion
Isoniazid	Tuberculosis	Depression, agitation, hallucinations, paranoia, impaired memory, anxiety
Lamivudine	HIV	Insomnia, mania
Methotrexate	Lymphoma	Encephalopathy (at high dose)
Pentamidine	*Pneumocystis carinii* pneumonia	Confusion, anxiety, lability, hallucinations
Procarbazine	Lymphoma	Mania, loss of appetite, insomnia, nightmares, confusion, malaise
Quinolones	Infection	Psychosis, delirium, seizures, anxiety, insomnia, depression
Stavudine	HIV	Headache, asthenia, malaise, confusion, depression, seizures, excitability, anxiety, mania, early morning awakening, insomnia
Sulfonamides	Infection	Psychosis, delirium, confusion, depression, hallucinations
Thiabendazole	Strongyloidiasis	Hallucinations, olfactory disturbance
Vinblastine	Kaposi sarcoma	Depression, loss of appetite, headache
Vincristine	Kaposi sarcoma	Hallucinations, headache, ataxia, sensory loss

(*continued*)

TABLE 12.3 (*continued*)

Drug	Target illness	Side-effects
Zalcitabine	HIV	Headaches, confusion, impaired concentration, somnolence, asthenia, depression, seizures, peripheral neuropathy
Zidovudine	HIV	Headache, malaise, asthenia, insomnia, unusually vivid dreams, restlessness, severe agitation, mania, auditory hallucinations, confusion

SUBSTANCE USE DISORDERS

Substance abuse is a comorbid disorder in many persons with HIV. Patients may present with intoxication, uncomplicated withdrawal, or withdrawal delirium. Psychosis or other psychiatric syndromes may also occur secondary to the substance use disorder.

DELIRIUM IN HIV

Delirium occurs frequently among HIV-infected patients and can result in agitation that requires emergency management. The etiology of delirium is often multifactorial in this group of patients, given the underlying HIV infection, the multiple medications such patients are often prescribed, and the frequency of the presence of multiple comorbid medical conditions such as infections, neoplasms, and metabolic disturbances. The risk of the occurrence of delirium is greater among those with HIV-related dementia. The clinical features of delirium in HIV cases are similar to those in other individuals not infected with HIV.

As in every case of delirium, the underlying medical cause must be identified and rapidly corrected. A detailed physical examination must be performed and the necessary investigations carried out. The drugs being taken by the patient need to be reviewed. The patient must be reoriented, and if necessary, low doses of antipsychotic medication can be used to manage the patient's behavior.

PSYCHOTROPIC EFFECTS OF HIV DRUGS

Psychosis, mania, agitation, and suicidal ideation are associated with antiretroviral treatment. The psychiatric symptoms most commonly occur within a month of commencing retroviral therapy, but the time of the onset of the symptoms can vary. These may resolve when the offending agent is discontinued; prophylactic agents can be used and may be continued for the next 1–3 months. Neuropsychiatric side-effects of selected medications used in HIV are given in Table 12.3.

CONCLUSION

In conclusion, the management of psychiatric emergencies among patients with medical conditions requires ensuring the patient's safety, identifying delirium and other medical etiologies, treating the underlying disorder, and providing symptomatic relief for the acute crisis with medication and psychological intervention. Appropriate plans must be made for the management of the patient after discharge.

REFERENCES

Battaglia, J, Moss, S, Rush, J, Kang, J, Mendoza, R, Leedom, L, Dubin, W, McGlynn, C and Goodman, L 1997, Haloperidol, lorazepam, or both for psychotic agitation? A multicenter, prospective, double-blind emergency department study. *Am J Emerg Med,* 15, 335–340.

Bennett, WR, Joesch, JM, Mazur, M and Roy-Byrne, P 2009, Characteristics of HIV-positive patients treated in a psychiatric emergency department. *Psychiatr Serv,* 60, 398–401.

Bieniek, SA, Ownby, RL, Penalver, A and Dominguez, RA 1998, A double-blind study of lorazepam versus the combination of haloperidol and lorazepam in managing agitation. *Pharmacotherapy,* 18, 57–62.

Breier, A, Meehan, K, Birkett, M, David, S, Ferchland, I, Sutton, V, Taylor, CC, Palmer, R, Dossenbach, M, Kiesler, G, Brook, S and Wright, P 2002, A double-blind, placebo-controlled dose-response comparison of intramuscular olanzapine and haloperidol in the treatment of acute agitation in schizophrenia. *Arch Gen Psychiatry,* 59, 441–448.

Chandra, PS, Desai, G and Ranjan, S 2005, HIV and psychiatric disorders. *Indian J Med Res,* 121, 451–467.

Cook, IA 2004, Guideline Watch: Practice Guideline for the Treatment of Patients with Delirium. Arlington, Va: American Psychiatric Association.

Gleason OC 2003, Delirium. *Am Fam Physician*, 67, 1027.

Halstead, S, Riccio, M, Harlow, P, Oretti, R and Thompson, C 1988, Psychosis associated with HIV infection. *Br J Psychiatry,* 153, 618–623.

Harris, MJ, Jeste, DV, Gleghorn, A and Sewell, DD 1991, New-onset psychosis in HIV-infected patients. *J Clin Psychiatry,* 52, 369–376.

Khouzam, HR, Tan, DT and Gill, TS 2007, *Handbook of emergency psychiatry*. Philadelphia: Elsevier.

McDaniel, JS, Brown, L, Cournos, F, Forstein, M, Goodkin, K, Lyketsos, C and Chung, JY 2010, *Practice guidelines for the treatment of patients with HIV/AIDS*. American Psychiatric Association.

Taylor, D, Paton, C and Kerwin, R 2007, *The Maudsley prescribing guidelines*. 9th ed. pp. 467–468. Informa Healthcare.

13 Psychiatric Emergencies in Personality Disorders

Ilyas Mirza, Atif Rahman

WHAT IS PERSONALITY DISORDER?

According to the International Classification of Diseases, 10th edition (ICD 10), a personality disorder is a severe disturbance in the characterological, constitutional, and behavioral tendencies of an individual, and usually involves several areas of the personality (WHO 1992). It is nearly always associated with considerable personal and social disruption. The disturbance is present for a good period of time. Personality disorders tend to appear in late childhood or adolescence and continue to manifest during adulthood. It is therefore unlikely that a diagnosis of personality disorder will be appropriate before the age of 16 or 17 years.

The areas of personality that are affected include (i) thinking, (ii) affect (immediate mood response), (iii) interpersonal functioning (relationships with friends, family, and colleagues at work), and (iv) impulse control (ability to control gratification).

Patients suffering from a personality disorder usually do not complain about the symptoms resulting from their disorder, unlike those with a mental illness, who do report their symptoms to a doctor. In the case of people with personality disorder, a lot of information has to be obtained from the family/caregiver. These patients usually present with problematic behaviors.

TYPES OF PERSONALITY DISORDERS

One useful way of classifying personality disorders is the DSM clustering system, which groups these disorders into broad clusters, as described below (Reich and Thompson 1987).

- *Cluster A – the odd or eccentric types:* Paranoid, schizoid, and schizotypal personality disorder
- *Cluster B – the dramatic, emotional or erratic types:* Histrionic, narcissistic, antisocial, and borderline personality disorders
- *Cluster C – the anxious and fearful types:* Obsessive–compulsive, avoidant, and dependent

This clustering system helps quantify the core elements of personality disorders in groups, which is useful when deciding on treatment and management in an emergency psychiatric setting.

In the emergency psychiatric setting, it is usually the cluster B personality disorders which attract the maximum attention. This is because they display poor impulse control and often present to the hospital in a crisis, threatening to harm either themselves or others.

Persons with cluster C personality disorders may also visit the hospital. They usually have acute psychosomatic complaints, which present a challenge in terms of their management.

It has been argued that personality dysfunction is best represented on a continuum or dimension, rather than categories. ICD 11 takes cognizance of this and defines personality dysfunction at different levels of severity ranging from no personality dysfunction to personality difficulty, mild, moderate, and severe personality disorder (Tyrer *et al.* 2011). The level of difficulty is then defined by description of the trait at the time of assessment including the recent past (*see* ICD 11 beta draft for descriptors http://apps.who.int/classifications/icd11/browse/l-m/en)

EPIDEMIOLOGY OF PERSONALITY DISORDERS

For long, it was believed that persons with personality disorders are found only in developed countries. Recent studies, however, indicate that these disorders are just as prevalent outside Europe, North America, and Australia (Tyrer *et al.* 2010c). The studies also highlight that problems in social functioning among people with personality disorder are clinically significant, even when the impact of other comorbid mental health problems has been controlled for. The estimates of prevalence are 6.1% (s.e. 0.3) for any personality disorder, and 3.6% (s.e. 0.3), 1.5% (s.e. 0.1) and 2.7% (s.e. 0.2) for clusters A, B, and C, respectively (Huang *et al.* 2009). The occurrence of personality disorders is significantly high among males, the previously married (Cluster C), the unemployed (Cluster C), the young (Clusters A and B), and the poorly educated. Personality disorders are highly comorbid with other mental illnesses. The impairments associated with personality disorders are only partially explained by comorbidity with mental or physical illnesses.

Individuals with personality disorders are more likely than others to suffer from alcohol and drug problems. In addition, they are more likely to experience adverse life events, such as difficulties in relationships, housing problems, and long-term unemployment.

DISSOCIAL/ANTI-SOCIAL PERSONALITY DISORDER

The most consistently studied personality disorder in community studies has been dissocial/antisocial personality disorder, the lifetime prevalence of which is between 2% and 3%. It is more commonly found to occur among men, younger people, those of low socioeconomic status, single individuals, the poorly educated, and those living in urban areas (Moran 1999). Persons with this disorder usually present through the criminal justice system.

Emotionally Unstable/Borderline Personality Disorder

This is generally the most prevalent (and certainly the most extensively researched) category in psychiatric settings. Patients with this disorder are regular users of psychiatric emergency services and utilize high levels of healthcare and social resources (Paris 2002). Although the crises in these cases are usually short-lived and resolve quickly, they tend to be severe. They are, therefore, often difficult to manage, and clinical and medicolegal complications may arise. An emergency psychiatrist needs to make two decisions concerning these patients: (i) whether hospitalization is required, and (ii) what medication, if any, should be prescribed (APA 2001).

The course of this disorder is quite variable. While the short-term outcomes are not too favorable, the results of long-term follow-up show that many patients ultimately cease to meet the criteria for this personality disorder. Nonetheless, the disorder can have serious consequences, with the reported suicide rate being 10% (Paris 2002). It is also very damaging in terms of the patient's quality of life, with recurrent losses of job, interrupted education, and broken marriages being commonly experienced. The condition is often misdiagnosed in adolescent patients due to the fact that their personalities are still developing.

CLINICAL FEATURES AND DIAGNOSIS

This chapter focuses on two of the cluster B disorders (dissocial/antisocial personality disorder and emotionally unstable/borderline personality disorder) as these are the most relevant to emergency psychiatric settings. Readers are advised to refer to ICD 10 or DSM-IV for the details of other disorders (WHO 1992; APA 2000).

The ICD-11, which is due to come out shortly, will contain for each personality disorder:

1. A definition, a set of inclusion and exclusion terms,
2. A description of the essential (required) features,
3. A characterization of the boundary of the disorder with normality (threshold for the diagnosis) and with other disorders (differential diagnosis),
4. A series of coded qualifiers/subtypes,
5. A description of course features, associated clinical presentations, culture-related features, developmental presentations, and gender-related features (Luciano 2015).

Emergency Presentations

Most of the presentations of personality disorders that one comes across in an emergency setting are a consequence of behavioral dyscontrol. There is a broad spectrum of symptoms, such as:

- Impulsive aggression
- Self-mutilation
- Psychosis-like symptoms, such as suspicious behavior, brief psychotic episodes, and delusional disorders
- Intense anger and depression.

CLUSTER B (DRAMATIC, EMOTIONAL, OR ERRATIC DISORDERS)

The distinctive features of the disorders which are included in this cluster are given below:

- *Dissocial/antisocial personality disorder:* A pervasive disregard for the law and the rights of others
- *Emotionally unstable/borderline personality disorder:* Instability in relationships, self-image, identity, and behavior, often leading to self-harm and impulsivity
- *Histrionic personality disorder:* Pervasive attention-seeking behavior, including inappropriate sexual seductiveness and shallow or exaggerated emotions
- *Narcissistic personality disorder:* A pervasive pattern of grandiosity, need for admiration, and a lack of empathy.

Those presenting in an emergency setting would have moderate to severe personality disorder.

Diagnostic Criteria with Case Vignettes

The problem of a person with dissocial/antisocial personality disorder usually comes to light because of a significant disparity between his behavior and the prevailing social norms (e.g. the spouse of a person with dissocial personality disorder may come to the emergency department (ED) with physical or emotional signs of repeated and severe domestic violence). The person's behavior is characterized by:

- Callous unconcern for the feelings of others
- A gross and persistent attitude of irresponsibility and disregard for social norms, rules, and obligations

BOX 13.1 A CASE

Mr X is a 24-year-old man who presented to the accident and emergency department following a road accident. He was drunk while driving and hit a lamp post. He initially denied that he had consumed alcohol and accused the hospital staff of tampering with the laboratory results. He then threatened the staff who had brought him to the hospital with violence if they reported the blood alcohol result to the police. The hospital staff called the police, who corroborated that Mr X was indeed intoxicated when they had arrested him. They also confirmed that he had a previous history of drunken driving, aggression, and theft. His partner reported that he had a history of violence and cruelty towards animals since early childhood.

Faced with this evidence, Mr X accepted that he had drunk alcohol before the accident, but blamed his circumstances for his predicament. He became very irritable and aggressive when the medical team suggested a treatment plan involving detoxification. He said that his partner drove him to drink and it was she who needed treatment rather than him.

BOX 13.2 A CASE

Miss Y is a 21-year-old woman who arrived in the emergency department after taking an overdose of 32 tablets of paracetmol. She was accompanied by her boyfriend, who reported that she had taken the overdose after an argument with him. He had told her that he planned to go for a vacation with his male friends. She got angry and accused him of not loving her.

On examining her, the hospital staff noticed superficial scarring on her forearms. When she was questioned further, she said she had been abused as a child. She said she had found it difficult to control her emotions and, in order to cope with the situation and release the psychological tension, had resorted to scratching her forearm superficially. She stated that she felt that her partner was abandoning her when he informed her that he planned a holiday with his friends. She could not cope with these feelings, became intensely angry, and took the overdose. She did not want to kill herself.

- Incapacity to maintain enduring relationships, though no difficulty is experienced in establishing them
- Very low tolerance to frustration and a low threshold for discharge of aggression, including violence
- Incapacity to experience guilt or to profit from experience, particularly punishment
- A marked tendency to blame others, or to offer plausible rationalizations, for the behavior that has brought the patient into conflict with society.

Persistent irritability may be present as an associated feature.

A person with an emotionally unstable personality disorder has a marked tendency to act impulsively without considering the consequences, and affective instability is also present. The ability to plan ahead may be minimal, and outbursts of intense anger often lead to violence or "behavioral explosions". These are easily precipitated when the person's impulsive (without planning) acts are criticized or thwarted by others.

BOX 13.3 A CASE

Miss Z came to the emergency department complaining of acute pain in the hand, accompanied by loss of function of the hand. The results of all the physical investigations were normal. When the hospital staff turned their attention to other patients, she began to sigh theatrically, as if she was having difficulty breathing. While she was being examined, she began to flirt with the doctor, telling him that she was sure that most of his female patients fell in love with him. As he explained to her that all her physical health parameters were normal, she began to pout and flutter her eyelashes seductively.

Her partner reported that she liked being the center of attention.

An example of a behavioral explosion is a young woman taking a drug overdose or committing a similar act of self-harm, such as superficial cutting.

The continuum of severity may vary from personality difficulties in an adolescence (coded as Z-non-disease entity to avoid stigmatization of those in transient adolescent crisis) to severe personality disorder.

Patients with *histrionic personality disorder* may come to the emergency room with dissociative/conversion symptoms. For example, a person may present with loss of hand function, which cannot be medically explained. There would be a history of:

- Self-dramatization, theatricality, exaggerated expression of emotions
- Suggestibility, being easily influenced by others or by circumstances
- Shallow and labile affectivity
- Continual search for excitement and activities in which the patient is the center of attention
- Inappropriate seductiveness in appearance or behavior
- Excessive concern about physical attractiveness.

A person with *narcissistic personality disorder* may be seen in an emergency setting when they come into conflict with the law or when they have been involved in problems related to interpersonal relations that result in physical health sequelae, such as injury. The personality of such a person is marked by a pervasive pattern of grandiosity (in fantasy or behavior), need for admiration and lack of empathy. These traits start to appear by early adulthood and can be manifested in a variety of ways. Five (or more) of the following manifestations must be present to make for a diagnosis of narcissistic personality disorder.

- Has a grandiose sense of self-importance (e.g. exaggerates achievements and talents, expects to be recognized as superior without commensurate achievements)
- Is preoccupied with fantasies of unlimited success, power, brilliance, beauty, or ideal love
- Believes that the individual is "special" and unique and can be understood only by, or should associate only with, other special or high-status people (or institutions)
- Requires excessive admiration
- Has a sense of entitlement, i.e. unreasonable expectations of especially favorable treatment or automatic compliance with his or her expectations
- Is interpersonally exploitative, i.e. takes advantage of others to achieve his/her own ends
- Lacks empathy: is unwilling to recognize or identify with the feelings and needs of others
- Is often envious of others or believes others are envious of him/her
- Displays arrogant, haughty behavior, or attitude.

INTERVIEWING AND EVALUATION

The general principles for taking the history of those with personality disorders are the same as those for any psychiatric disorder. However, further exploration is usually required through the use of key questions that may indicate the presence of a cluster B personality disorder. A functional assessment is also necessary. Very often, a lot of probing is required since some persons with personality disorder are not very forthcoming about their problems.

The general principles for taking the history include listing of the patient's current problems and what has precipitated them. The latter helps to clarify why the person is presenting now. Information is obtained from the patient, relatives or case notes, if available, to find out whether the current presentation is similar to a previous presentation, and if so, what treatment had helped at that time. Particular attention should be paid to obtaining a previous history of self-harm. This should be done in a sensitive and non-judgmental manner. If the patient has come to the ED in a crisis, then one needs to identify any previous crises and how they were dealt with. The social history, including a change in social circumstances, and the presence of substance use may provide clues to the current presentation.

The answers to a few specific key questions may indicate the presence of cluster B personality disorders. These are:

- Are you a person whose mood goes up and down?
- Do you lose your temper easily?
- Do you like being in the center of things?
- Do you often act on impulse?

Gunn (1993) emphasizes that for practical clinical purposes, the most useful approach is to undertake a functional assessment of the personality. This helps make the clinician and patient draw a link between the distress and the disability in functioning; it thus makes it easier to draw up a clinical management plan. According to Gunn, developing a functional assessment involves three main tasks. First, one must list the abnormal features of the personality in relation to:

- Thinking, the patients' beliefs about themselves (e.g. low self-esteem, a sense of entitlement out of proportion to the situation) and their beliefs about others (e.g. everyone is hostile and untrustworthy)
- Feelings and emotions, any abnormalities in the quality or intensity of emotions, such as outbursts of inappropriate anger, rapidly fluctuating mood, persistent low mood, anxiety, low tolerance, or frustration
- Behavior
- Interpersonal functioning, interpersonal problems such as the inability to trust others and the tendency to invite rejection, to become dependent or to form unstable intense relationships
- Insight.

Second, one must describe the associated distress in terms of mental illnesses, such as clinical syndromes of depression, substance misuse, psychosis or anxiety, or more non-specific physical or psychological symptoms. Third, quantify associated interference with functioning in terms of family functioning (including functioning in relation to partner and to children), social (housing, finance, social relationships, crime), and occupational.

This will enable the clinician to understand the social context of the patient, and elucidate the precipitating, perpetuating and predisposing factors, as is done in the assessment of other mental disorders.

As stated at the beginning of this chapter, defining personality disorder according to severity is a major shift of emphasis with regard to evaluation and is consistent with developing an enabling and recovery-oriented classificatory system.

MANAGEMENT

Bateman and Tyrer (2002) defined certain principles for the treatment of personality disorders. They stated that the treatment should:

- be well-structured
- have a clear focus
- have a theoretical basis that is coherent both to the staff and the patient
- be relatively long-term
- be well-integrated with other services or resources available to the patient
- involve a clear treatment alliance between the staff and the patient.

The most important factor is to have explicit and realistic goals, which, in the emergency psychiatric setting, would be support, monitoring and supervision, intervening in crises, increasing the patients' motivation and compliance, improving their understanding of difficulties, building a therapeutic relationship, avoiding deterioration, limiting harm through short-term interventions in specific areas such as anger, self-harm, social skills, and offending behavior, and linking with the patient through long-term follow-up and support (Davison 2002). Sometimes, giving the patient practical advice on and support in areas such as housing, finance, and childcare can contain a crisis. It may not be possible to stabilize the person to the baseline level of functioning in one session.

Inpatient admission should be considered to prevent further harm and reduce the risk of suicide, and to facilitate the treatment of comorbid psychosis or severe depression (Fagin 2004). It may also be indicated if the patient displays very chaotic behavior that endangers them. However, a person should be admitted only if the unit has the capacity, in terms of skills, staffing and clinical pressures, to manage the patient.

DRUGS, PSYCHOLOGICAL, AND SOCIAL TREATMENTS

Psychosocial treatment is the treatment of choice for the management of personality disorders. However, these patients usually present in an emergency setting, where the immediate distress can be effectively relieved by appropriate pharmacotherapy, together with social intervention. These modalities help to reduce the risk of harm to the self or others.

The social interventions that can assist in managing personality disorders in an emergency setting include enlisting the support of the patient's family/peers in helping with self-management during a crisis, and the use of legal instruments such as probation orders if there is offending behavior to ensure that the patient attends treatment programs (drug, alcohol, or psychosocial).

Antipsychotics can be used for the treatment of cognitive/perceptual symptoms, such as suspiciousness, paranoid ideation, ideas of reference, odd communication, muddled thinking, magical thinking, episodic distortions of reality, derealization, depersonalization, illusions, and stress-induced hallucinations (Tyrer and Bateman 2004b).

Selective serotonin reuptake inhibitors (SSRIs) are useful in controlling symptoms of affective dysregulation, such as lability of mood, "rejection sensitivity", mood crashes, inappropriate intense anger, outbursts of temper, chronic emptiness, dysphoria, loneliness, inability to experience pleasure, and social anxiety and avoidance.

Mood stabilizers and SSRIs can be helpful in controlling impulsive-behavioral dyscontrol, which may manifest itself as sensation-seeking, risky or reckless behavior, no reflective delay, low tolerance of frustration, impulsive aggression, recurrent assaultiveness, making threats, destruction of property, impulsive binges (drugs, alcohol, food, sex, spending), recurrent suicidal threats and behavior, and self-mutilation.

As for psychological treatments, it is usually not practical or recommended to deliver these interventions in an emergency setting (Tyrer and Bateman 2004a). It may, however, be useful to suggest the use of therapies such as cognitive behavior therapy (to alter dysfunctional core beliefs), and dialectical behavior therapy (initially, to reduce self-harm; eventually, to achieve transcendence) to the patient and the treating team. Recent evidence also shows that cognitive–analytic therapy (to achieve greater self-understanding), behavior therapy (to improve maladaptive behavior) and nidotherapy (to achieve better environmental adjustment, thus minimizing the impact of the disorder) are effective to some extent.

A psychological intervention that may be possible in an emergency setting is conducting a therapeutic interview based on the principles of assessment and management described above. Such an interview might have the effect of making the patient feel that they are understood, and thus help to contain, manage, and process the intense feelings that might have precipitated the crisis.

CONCLUSION

Patients with personality disorders may present to the emergency setting in a crisis. Evaluation reveals a long-standing pattern of relating to oneself and the environment. It is helpful to quantify severity of the presentation along with description of the problems in order to formulate a coherent treatment plan and to monitor progress. The treatment is usually long-term and psychosocial in nature. The immediate interventions in the emergency setting are aimed at minimizing harm and guiding the patient towards the appropriate long-term treatment. The therapeutic interview, social interventions, and the judicious use of psychotropic drugs help contain the crisis and thus prevent deterioration.

REFERENCES

American Psychiatric Association (APA) 2000, *Diagnostic and Statistical Manual of Mental Disorders*. 4th edition, Text Revision (DSM-IV-TR). Washington DC: APA.

American Psychiatric Association (APA) 2001, Practice guideline for the treatment of patients with borderline personality disorder. *Am J Psychiatry,* 158, 1–52.

Bateman, A and Tyrer, P 2002, Effective management of personality disorder. Available at http://www.dh.gov.uk/prod_consum_dh/groups/dh_digitalassets/@dh/@en/documents/digitalasset/dh_4130843.pdf

Davison, S 2002, Principles of managing patients with personality disorder. *Adv Psychiatr Treat,* 8, 1–9.

Fagin, L 2004, Management of personality disorders in acute in-patient settings. Part 1: Borderline personality disorders. *Adv Psychiatr Treat,* 10, 93–99.

Gunn, J 1993, Personality disorders. In: Gunn, J and Taylor, P (eds). *Forensic psychiatry: Clinical, legal and ethical issues*, pp. 373–406. London: Butterworth Heinemann.

Huang, Y, Kotov, R, de Girolamo, G, Preti, A, Angermeyer, M, Benjet, C, Demyttenaere, K, Graaf, R, Gureje, O, Karam, A, Lee, S, Lépine, JP, Matschinger, H, Posada-Villa, J, Suliman, S, Vilagut, G and Kessler, R 2009, DSM-IV personality disorders in the WHO World Mental Health Surveys. *Br J Psychiatry,* 195, 46–53.

Luciano, M 2015, The ICD-11 beta draft is available online. *World Psychiatry* 14, 375–376. Published online 2015 September 25. doi: 10.1002/wps.20262.

Moran, P 1999, The epidemiology of antisocial personality disorder. *Soc Psychiatry Psychiatr Epidemiol,* 34, 231–242.

Paris, J 2002, Implications of long-term outcome research for the management of patients with borderline personality disorder. *Harv Rev Psychiatry,* 10, 315–323.

Reich, J and Thompson, W 1987, DSM-III personality disorder clusters in three populations. *Br J Psychiatry,* 50, 471–475.

Tyrer, P and Bateman, A 2004a, Psychological treatment for personality disorders. *Adv Psychiatr Treat,* 10, 378–388.

Tyrer, P and Bateman, A 2004b, Drug treatment for personality disorders. *Adv Psychiatr Treat,* 10, 389–398.

Tyrer, P, Mulder, R, Crawford, M, Newton-Howes, G, Simonsen, E, Ndetei, D, Koldobsky, N, Fossati, A, Mbatia, J and Barrett, B 2010, Personality disorder: A new global perspective. *World Psychiatry,* 9, 56–60.

Tyrer, P, Crawford, M, Mulder, R, Blashfield, R, Farnam, A and Fossati, A 2011, The rationale for the reclassification of personality disorder in the 11th Revision of the International Classification of Diseases. *Personal Ment Health,* 5, 246–259.

World Health Organization (WHO) 1992, *International Classification of Diseases*, 10th edition. Geneva: WHO.

14 Legal Aspects of Psychiatric Emergencies

Parmanand Kulhara, Sandeep Grover

INTRODUCTION

Psychiatric emergencies are defined as acute disturbances of thought, mood, or behavior that require immediate intervention (Barton 1983). The response to a psychiatric emergency depends on the country and the resources available, and draws upon a support system that includes caregivers, the therapist, the family doctor, the police, a mobile team, the emergency room, and the insurance company or managed care organization (Breslow 2002). Depending on the country and the policy of the hospital, three basic models have been described for the delivery of emergency psychiatry services: (i) the psychiatrist sees the patient in the medical emergency department (ED); (ii) the psychiatrist sees the patient in the medical ED but in a separate section, where specially trained and dedicated staff is available to deal with mentally ill patients; and (iii) stand-alone psychiatry emergency services for acutely mentally ill patients (Zeller 2010). In a resource-poor country such as India, it is the first model which applies in the case of most psychiatry emergency services.

LEGAL ASPECTS OF PSYCHIATRIC EMERGENCIES

The important legal aspects that confront a mental health professional while dealing with psychiatric emergencies are obtaining consent for treatment and involuntary admission of the patient.

The general norm is that mentally ill patients should be treated with their consent as they have the right to choose a treatment on the assumption that they have insight (they recognize that they have an illness) and good judgment (they know that they can get help from psychiatric service providers) (Andreasen and Black 2000). However, not all patients brought to the hospital with psychiatric emergencies readily agree to get themselves treated and admitted. In such a situation, depending on the law of the land, the psychiatrist has to go against the will of the patient while making a decision on the issues of treatment and admission. In legal terms, such admissions are understood as involuntary hospitalization/admission and are based on the assessment that the person is mentally ill and a danger to himself or others (Habib, van Rooyen and Hiemstra 2007; Simon and Shuman 2007). With the new Clinical Establishment Act, 2010 (The Gazette of India, Clinial Establishments [Registration and Regulation] Act 2010), it is important to remember that treatment facility must be registered with the government as per the rules.

INVOLUNTARY HOSPITALIZATION/ ADMISSION

One should resort to involuntary hospitalization/admission only as an emergency psychiatric intervention, when other less restrictive means of treatment are not appropriate (Simon and Goetz 1999). Usually, involuntary admission is warranted when the patients' behavior poses a danger to their life (e.g. a suicidal patient) or to that of others (e.g. a homicidal and/or violent patient), or if patients are in such a state that they cannot look after their basic needs. The indications for involuntary admission are listed in Table 14.1.

However, while making a decision on involuntary hospitalization, the psychiatrist has to cautiously balance the risk–benefit ratio, i.e. the decision should not infringe on the civil rights of the patient or others and at the same time, it should take into account the risk of self-harm or harm to others. It is to be remembered that involuntary hospitalization should be based on clinical judgment and not on societal needs. An effort should be made to deal with the patient with empathy and to explain why they are being admitted against their will. Family members, if available, should be involved in the decision-making process to reduce the trauma of involuntary admission (Simon and Shuman 2007).

In India, the Mental Health Act, 1987 (MHA 1987) governs involuntary admissions (MHA 1987). Chapter IV of the MHA, 1987 deals with admission and detention in psychiatric hospitals or nursing homes. The MHA, 1987 does not provide specific provisions for involuntary admission in emergency situations, but some of the provisions of the Act can be used for involuntary admission or voluntary admission of minors in the emergency set-up.

In case the minor patients (less than 18 years of age) are brought to the psychiatric ED, they can be admitted if their guardian considers them to be a mentally ill person and desires to admit them in any psychiatric hospital or psychiatric nursing home for treatment. The guardian may request the medical officer-in-charge to admit the minor as a voluntary patient. Part II of Chapter IV of the MHA, 1987 discusses the subject of admission in special circumstances and according to its provisions, "Any mentally ill person who does not, or is unable to, express his willingness for admission as a

TABLE 14.1

Indications for Involuntary Admission to a Hospital

- Poses danger to himself (e.g. suicidal patient)
- Poses danger to others (e.g. homicidal, violent patient)
- Is unable to look after his basic needs (e.g. gravely disabled patient)
- Poses danger to property
- Lacks capacity to make rational treatment decisions

Source: Simon and Shuman 2007; Simon and Goetz 1999

voluntary patient, may be admitted and kept as an inpatient in a psychiatric nursing hospital or psychiatric nursing home on an application made in that behalf by a relative or a friend of the mentally ill person if the medical officer-in-charge is satisfied that in the interest of the mentally ill person it is necessary to do so." Further, the Act states: "Every application under subsection shall be in the prescribed form and be accompanied by two medical certificates, from two medical practitioners of whom one shall be a medical practitioner in the service of Government, to the effect that the condition of such mentally ill person is such that he should be kept under observation and treatment as an inpatient in a psychiatric hospital or psychiatric nursing home." Alternatively, the medical officer-in-charge of the psychiatric hospital or psychiatric nursing home concerned may, if satisfied that it is proper to do so, cause a mentally ill person to be examined by two medical practitioners (working in the hospital or in the nursing home) instead of requiring such certificates.

Part III of Chapter IV of the MHA, 1987 deals with the reception order, which can be made by the medical officer-in-charge of a psychiatric hospital or psychiatric nursing home, or by the spouse or any other relative of the mentally ill person. A person may be admitted against their will if "the medical officer-in-charge of a psychiatric hospital or psychiatric nursing home in which a mentally ill person is undergoing treatment under a temporary treatment order is satisfied that the mentally ill person is suffering from mental disorder of such a nature and degree that his treatment in the psychiatric hospital or as the case may be, psychiatric nursing home, is required to be continued for more than six months, or it is necessary in the interests of the health and personal safety of the mentally ill person or for the protection of others that such person shall be detained in a psychiatric hospital or psychiatric nursing home." This provision can be used in the emergency setting to secure an involuntary admission. Under the Act, a medical officer-in-charge who is in favor of an involuntary admission can make an application to the magistrate under whose jurisdiction the psychiatric hospital or psychiatric nursing home falls, seeking the detention of the mentally ill person in the psychiatric hospital or psychiatric nursing home under a reception order.

Alternatively, "The husband or wife of a person who is alleged to be mentally ill or, where there is no husband or wife, or where the husband or wife is prevented by reason of any illness or absence from India or otherwise from making the application, any other relative of such person may make an application to the magistrate within the local limits of whose jurisdiction the said person ordinarily resides, for the detention of the alleged mentally ill person under a reception order in a psychiatric hospital or psychiatric nursing home" (MHA 1987).

It is to be remembered that the application must be made in the prescribed form and should be signed and verified in the prescribed manner. It should state whether any previous application has been made to inquire into the mental condition of the allegedly mentally ill person. The application should be accompanied by two medical certificates from two medical practitioners, of whom one must be a medical practitioner in the service of the government.

As is clear from the above, the MHA, 1987 is silent on the issue of what to do in the emergency set-up if a patient refuses admission and the clinician feels that admission is necessary because the patient's life or the life of others is at risk. The only saving grace is that in India, the patient is most often brought to the ED by their relatives or guardian. Hence, in case the patient refuses admission but the clinician feels that admission is the best option, the patient can be admitted under the provision stipulating that the family members can give the medical officer-in-charge an application seeking admission. Alternatively, the patient can be admitted after being examined by two medical practitioners working in the hospital or nursing home instead of requiring such certificates.

INFORMED CONSENT

The basic tenet of medical ethics is to respect the autonomy of the individual. From the ethical point of view, it is considered that every person has the capacity and right to make decisions about their own healthcare. Informed consent is not only a legal and ethical requirement, good clinical practice also suggests that it should be obtained from all patients before they are started on treatment. Obtaining informed consent strengthens the therapeutic alliance between the psychiatrist and the patient, and also protects the psychiatrist from legal complications, such as the patient or family members later alleging negligence or accusing the psychiatrist of administering treatment for which no valid informed consent was obtained (Simon and Goetz 1999). The clinician should remember that administering treatment without the consent or against the will of the patient may constitute battery and commencing treatment without adequate consent is considered an act of medical negligence (Simon and Shuman 2007).

The question of who should obtain informed consent is an important one. It is the treating psychiatrist who must do so as it is considered insufficient if the consent is obtained by the nurse or other healthcare professionals who are a part of the treating team. Psychiatrists are usually best equipped to answer the patient's questions about the proposed treatment.

It is well-known that many mentally ill persons are not competent to make decisions on their treatment because of their altered mental state or disturbances in their cognitive ability (Simon and Shuman 2007). However, it must be understood that refusal to consent is not equivalent to incompetence. It is also important to remember that lack of insight does not preclude obtaining informed consent, because many psychotic patients are capable of giving valid consent for treatment. On the other hand, psychiatrists should also be aware of the fact that many patients may consent to treatment although they do not understand the consequences of such treatment. In such situation, consent should be obtained from the patient's relatives.

The main points to be remembered about informed consent in a psychiatric emergency set-up are given in Table 14.2. In an emergency situation, 'competence' is understood as the patient's ability to understand the particular treatment option being proposed, make a treatment choice and verbally or non-verbally communicate that choice to the treating psychiatrist (Simon and Goetz 1999).

Treatment should not be withheld as a result of the patient's lack of capacity to make a decision on their healthcare. What is required in such situations is obtaining consent from a key relative. In an emergency situation in which non-consenting patients

TABLE 14.2

Points to Remember about Informed Consent

- The three basic components of informed consent are competency, information, and volunatariness.
- Consent should be seen as a process rather than a single ritualistic event.
- Consent must be obtained by the treating psychiatrist rather than other members of the treating team.
- All details should be documented properly.
- If the patient is not able to give consent, then it should be obtained from a relative and this should be properly documented.
- In the case of minors and those considered to be incompetent, consent must be obtained from the guardian.

pose a danger to themselves or others, an exception may be made and they may be treated without informed consent. However, in this kind of a scenario, care should be taken to properly document the details of the situation which necessitated such a decision. The important thing to note is that "emergency" is determined on the basis of the patient's condition and on the basis of adverse circumstances. In this regard it is important to remember that patients have the right to ask for their treatment records under the Right to Information Act (The Gazette of India, Right to Information Act 2005). Hence, it is important to document as to how lack of capacity was established and who gave the consent on behalf of the patient for the involuntary treatment.

If the patient is a minor or disabled, the law generally allows the clinician to obtain informed consent from the patient's key relatives or legal guardian.

The other important legal and ethical issues to be kept in mind in the emergency setting are those of therapeutic privilege and waiver. Therapeutic privilege allows the treating psychiatrist to withhold certain information, the disclosure of which might have a serious, detrimental effect on the patient's physical and psychological health. However, it is important to understand that therapeutic privilege cannot be invoked if it is felt that providing information may cause the patient to reject treatment. It is recommended that therapeutic privilege be invoked only when it is clear that the disclosure of the information might cause the patient to become so alarmed that his decision-making abilities are disrupted. Waiver refers to a situation in which a patient who is competent knowingly and voluntarily waives the right to information on the treatment he is going to receive. If such is the case, the patient's decision to waive the right to information should be documented properly. However, it is important to remember that Indian laws are silent on these situations and these issues may not be admissible in a court of law.

Chapter VIII of the MHA, 1987 discusses the issue of consent, i.e. protection of the human rights of mentally ill persons. According to the Act, "No mentally ill person shall be subjected during treatment to any indignity (whether physical or mental) or cruelty; no mentally ill person under treatment shall be used for purposes of research, unless such research is of direct benefit to him for purposes of diagnosis or treatment, or such person, being a voluntary patient, has given his consent in writing or where such person (whether or not a voluntary patient) is incompetent, by reason of minority or otherwise, to give valid consent, the guardian or other person competent to give consent on his behalf has given his consent in writing for such research" (MHA 1987).

Issues related to the consent of persons with mental retardation are dealt with in the National Trust Act, 1999 (Mental Retardation and Multiple Disabilities Act 1999), which allows the appointment of a guardian who is to take all legal decisions on behalf of the person. Hence, while dealing with persons with mental retardation in emergency situations, the psychiatrist should enquire about the patient's legal guardian and seek their consent for treatment, including various procedures, and hospitalization.

The MHA, 1987 provides basic guidelines on how to handle issues related to the mentally ill. However, it is silent on the issue of consent for treatment, although it discusses the issues of consent for research and involuntary admission (discussed in another section). It should be appreciated that this silence also means that mentally ill persons have the same human rights as mentally sound persons and other laws governing these issues are also applicable to mentally ill persons. Chapter IV, section 16 of the MHA, 1987 empowers the mentally ill patient's family members to get them admitted to and treated in a psychiatric set-up. Hence, in case there is a need to admit a patient involuntarily and they are not able to provide informed consent, consent should be obtained from the family members.

SECLUSION AND RESTRAINT

In certain psychiatric emergencies, the psychiatrist may be left with no choice but to seclude and restrain the patient. In many cases, when patients improve and understand their clinical condition, they are grateful to the treating team for secluding and/or restraining them. However, there are situations in which the patient, after improving, feels that their basic human rights have been violated and they may seek legal redressal. Hence, it is important for clinicians to have some knowledge of the legal aspects of seclusion and restraint.

Seclusion is understood as involuntary confinement of a person alone in a room, which they are is physically prevented from leaving, or separating the patient from others and placing them in a safe, contained, controlled environment. Restraint is understood as the direct application of physical force to an individual, with or without their permission, to restrict their freedom of movement. Physical force may be applied through human touch, mechanical devices, or a combination of these. Some authors also include the use of drugs in the definition of restraint (Simon and Shuman 2007).

Unfortunately, in almost all treatment settings in India, there is no place available to seclude the patient. Hence, in emergency situations in which no other options are available, patients are restrained chemically or physically. It is also unfortunate that the MHA, 1987 does not specify anything clearly about physical restraint. It suggests that whenever it is felt that restraint is the best option available to ensure the safety of the patient or others, the need for restraint should be explained to the patient and informed consent for restraint must be obtained from them. Further, whenever a patient is restrained, it should be done for a minimal duration of time. As in the case of informed consent, some clinicians consider that the subject of applying restraint can be viewed as being covered under Chapter IV of the MHA, 1987, which discusses admission in special situations. As this chapter authorizes the family members to get the patient admitted to a hospital, some clinicians feel that the consent of family members may be sufficient and valid in the matter of restraint as well.

Restraint should never be used as a punishment or for the convenience of the treating team. Further, a patient who has been restrained should be monitored carefully by the clinician and/or other staff from time to time (at intervals of about 15 minutes), and the restraints should be removed at the earliest, after considering the risk–benefit ratio (Simon and Shuman 2007). Also, proper documentation of the clinical situation in which restraint was considered is necessary. Similarly, the reasons for the continuation of restraint must be documented.

CONFIDENTIALITY

The general rules of confidentiality guiding other aspects of psychiatry apply to psychiatric emergencies too. The treating psychiatrist is not expected to share with others the information provided to them by the patient in confidence, unless it is necessary for the treatment of the patient or in situations which call for exceptions to confidentiality (e.g. disclosure of information in the court).

CONCLUSION

With the increasing deinstitutionalization of mentally ill patients, most of these patients are managed in the community. However, because of the chronic or relapsing course of major psychiatric disorders, many patients experience exacerbation of their illness and visit the emergency services of hospitals, requiring short-term or long-term admission and treatment. Hence, physicians and psychiatrists working in the emergency set-up should be aware of the legal issues involved in dealing with these patients in emergency situations. Whenever possible, informed consent for treatment must be obtained from patients and if they require hospitalization, voluntary admission must be encouraged. When this is not possible, informed consent for treatment and hospitalization must be obtained from their relatives. As the condition of the patient stabilizes, an attempt should be made to convert involuntary admission to voluntary admission and the patient should be involved in all treatment decisions.

REFERENCES

Andreasen, C and Black, DW 2000, *Introductory textbook of psychiatry*. 3rd ed. pp. 667–71. Arlington VA: American Psychiatric Publishing Inc.

Barton, GM 1983, *Task force report on psychiatric emergency care issues*. Washington DC: American Psychiatric Association.

Breslow, RE 2002, Structure and function of psychiatric emergency services. In: Allen, MH (ed). *Emergency psychiatry*. Washington DC: American Psychiatric Publishing Inc.

Habib, T, van Rooyen, FC and Hiemstra, LA 2007, Involuntary admission of psychiatric patients in the Northern Cape Province and the accuracy of the initial psychiatric assessment done by the referring general practitioners. *S Afr Fam Pract,* 49, 14.

Mental Health Act (MHA) 1987, Government of India.

Mental Retardation and Multiple Disabilities Act 1999, National Trust for Welfare of Persons with Autism, Cerebral Palsy, Ministry of Law, Justice and Company Affairs, Government of India.

Simon, RI and Goetz, S 1999, Forensic issues in the psychiatric emergency department. *Psychiatr Clin North Am,* 22, 851–864.

Simon, RI and Shuman, DW 2007, Involuntary admission. In: Simon, RI, Shuman, DW and Arlington, D (eds). *Clinical manual of psychiatry and law.* Washington DC: American Psychiatric Publishing Inc.

The Gazette of India, Clinial Establishments (Registration and Regulation) Act 2010. Ministry of Law and Justice. New Delhi, Aug 19, 2010. No. 31.

The Gazette of India, Right to Information Act 2005. Ministry of Law and Justice. New Delhi, Act No. 22 of 2005, modified 2011.

Zeller, SL 2010, Treatment of psychiatric patients in emergency settings. *Primary Psychiatry,* 17, 35–41.

15 Psychiatric Emergencies in the Elderly

Sumesh T.P., Shaji K.S.

The diagnosis and management of behavioral disorders occurring late in life can be challenging. In the case of older people, one frequently comes across problems of comorbidity and issues related to the tolerability and adverse effects of medications. When psychiatric symptoms appear for the first time in late life, underlying physical and organic causes need to be considered, and a complete physical and neurological examination is mandatory. The causes for the symptoms are usually multiple and laboratory investigations may be required to pinpoint them.

There are many situations in which an immediate psychiatric assessment will help in managing the problems of the elderly. Proper evaluation and careful management can improve the outcome. The following are some of the problems the elderly can present with:

- Agitation or aggressive behavior
- Sudden change in behavior/personality
- Hallucinations/illusions of a sudden onset
- Suspiciousness/delusional thinking
- Disorientation/memory problems
- Fearfulness/anxiety of a sudden onset
- Sleep-related problems
- Problems related to alcohol/substance abuse
- Suicidal behavior.

Many psychiatric syndromes could lead to the symptoms mentioned above. However, as mentioned earlier, when psychiatric symptoms appear for the first time in late life, underlying physical or organic causes are to be considered. What appears to be psychiatric disease could very well be organic in etiology. Psychiatric evaluation of an older person in an emergency department (ED) should always include a thorough medical and neurological evaluation. The evaluation should lead to a tentative diagnosis and a management plan should be drawn up. The patient should then be closely monitored. Periodic review and interaction with those involved in the care of the patient will help.

Common psychiatric emergencies in the elderly (older than 65 years) may be considered under the following subheadings:

- Delirium
  - Delirium without dementia
  - Delirium with dementia
  - Delirium in alcohol withdrawal state
- Behavioral and psychological symptoms of dementia (BPSD)
- Psychosis
- Depression and suicidal behavior
- Anxiety disorders.

This chapter focuses on conditions for which urgent psychiatric consultation is needed. During the consultation, the clinician should carefully look for evidence of cognitive disorder, which is very common among this age group. The patient's spouse or caregiver will be able to throw light on whether the patient has been having difficulties in attention/concentration recently, or whether there has been any disorientation to time and/or place. Cognitive disturbance is usually more evident at night. Fluctuations in the level of consciousness are common. There could be periods of clear sensorium in between.

DELIRIUM

Delirium or an acute confusional state is common among older people and constitutes a medical emergency. It is caused by a transient, usually reversible, cerebral dysfunction, and is characterized by clouding of the consciousness. Delirium should be considered as the first possibility whenever an older person presents with behavioral problems that are sudden in onset. It is treatable and reversible if detected early, but the identification of the cause/causes is critical for prompt management (Khurana, Gambhir and Kishore 2011). Unidentified, unmanaged delirium can later on lead to other problems (Heymann *et al.* 2010). Delay makes it even more difficult to recognize the signs and symptoms of the disease which is causing the delirium. It can also lead to a disruption of the clinical care environment, cause physical injury to the patient, caregivers, and healthcare professionals, adversely affect the quality of care for the patient and prolong his stay in the hospital. Untreated delirium is associated with increased morbidity and mortality. Patients who develop delirium during hospitalization have a high mortality rate while in the hospital and during the months following discharge (Han *et al.* 2010). Delirium is one of the most common causes of behavioral problems among the elderly in the general medical, surgical, and postoperative wards.

The diagnosis of delirium is always clinical and no specific laboratory test is needed for its diagnosis. The diagnosis remains valid even if the investigations fail to identify any cause. The patient is often unable to provide accurate information. Gathering information from the caregivers can help identify the cause.

Clinical Features

- Clouding of consciousness
- Difficulty maintaining or shifting attention
- Disorientation

- Illusions
- Hallucinations
- Fluctuating levels of consciousness – the symptoms tend to fluctuate over the course of the day, with some improvement in the daytime and the maximum disturbance at night
- Reversal of the sleep–wake cycle
- Neurological symptoms such as dysphasia, dysarthria, and tremors
- Asterixis in hepatic encephalopathy and uremia.

Risk Factors

- Advanced age (especially above 80 years)
- Severe illness (especially cancer)
- Dehydration
- Dementia
- Fever
- Substance abuse
- Abnormal sodium levels
- Polypharmacy
- Visual or hearing impairment.

We may subdivide delirium in the elderly into three subgroups for ease of understanding and to facilitate its management:

- Delirium without dementia
- Delirium superimposed on dementia
- Delirium secondary to alcohol withdrawal.

Delirium without Dementia

There may be multiple causes for the occurrence of delirium in an older person who does not have a pre-existing cognitive disorder. Aging predisposes a person to the development of delirium.

Common Causes

- Infections
  - Pneumonia
  - Urinary tract infections
  - Central nervous system infections
- Metabolic abnormalities
  - Electrolyte imbalance
  - Hypoxia
  - Hypoglycemia
  - Hepatic or renal failure
  - Vitamin deficiency states (especially thiamine and cyanocobalamin)
- Structural lesions of the brain
  - Cerebrovascular events: Cerebral infarcts, subarachnoid hemorrhage

  - Primary or metastatic tumors
  - Brain abscess
- Toxic causes
  - Substance intoxication and withdrawal – alcohol, benzodiazepines
  - Anticholinergics (antihistamines, tricyclic antidepressants)
  - Anti-Parkinson drugs (levodopa)
- Hypoperfusion states
  - Shock
  - Cardiac arrhythmias
- Miscellaneous causes.

Sensory deprivation, sleep deprivation, fecal impaction, urinary retention, a change of environment, the use of physical restraints or of a bladder catheter, malnutrition and postictal state can also cause delirium. Delirium is most often multifactorial in etiology. This is particularly so in the case of the elderly. Multiple causes need to be considered in every case and the management of the patient should include correction of all the abnormalities detected.

Delirium with Dementia

Pre-existing dementia is a strong risk factor for the development of delirium in older people. Patients with undetected dementia can present to emergency services with superimposed delirium. The diagnosis becomes difficult when both delirium and dementia coexist and the more so, when the delirium is of the hypoactive type. The distinguishing feature is the impaired state of consciousness. One needs to ascertain whether there has been a history of cognitive decline and of the presence of clinical features suggestive of dementia in the preceding months. Recent exacerbation of behavioral symptoms accompanied by sleep disturbance would indicate the onset of superimposed delirium. In such situations, both conditions can be diagnosed.

Delirium Secondary to Alcohol Withdrawal

Older people may present to the emergency room with delirium caused by alcohol withdrawal. The diagnosis is easier when there is a temporal correlation between the onset of delirium and abstinence from alcohol. However, the fact that medical illnesses are very common among this age group makes the diagnosis difficult. Delirium due to alcohol withdrawal can be complicated by medical conditions, which can cause delirium. Evaluation for comorbid medical conditions is mandatory even when the clinical features are very suggestive of delirium tremens.

Investigations

Investigations are essential for the identification and management of the primary etiological factors. Depending on the clinical situation, the investigations might include a full blood count, blood sugar level, liver function tests, renal function tests, thyroid function test, urine analysis, ECG, EEG, lumbar puncture, and imaging studies (chest X-ray, CT scan, or MRI scan of the brain).

Management of Delirium

General Principles

The goals of the management of a patient with delirium are to identify the causes of the delirium and control the behavioral disturbance, if any. Paying attention to all possible causes will aid the patient's recovery. The management strategies are:

- Pharmacological
- Non-pharmacological
- Concerned with the prevention of complications.

Pharmacological Management

The short-term use of antipsychotics remains the treatment of choice for the control of behavioral symptoms. The pharmacological management of elderly patients with delirium is similar to that of younger patients, except that one should start with lower doses. Haloperidol is widely used for the control of restlessness and agitation (Leentjens and van der Mast 2005). To keep the behavioral symptoms under control intravenous administration is recommended of 0.25–0.5 mg of haloperidol every 8 hours on a scheduled basis and 0.25–0.5 mg every 6 hours, as needed. If oral dosing is used, then a higher dose, of 0.5–1.0 mg every 8 hours on a scheduled basis or 0.5–1.0 mg every 6 hours, as needed, would be helpful. Once the symptoms are controlled, the dose can be reduced or discontinued over a period of 3–5 days or earlier. Using the suggested low doses minimizes the risk of QTc prolongation. A baseline ECG may be taken and if the QTc interval is more than 450 milliseconds, haloperidol has to be avoided. Atypical antipsychotics such as risperidone, quetiapine, or olanzapine can also be used. They are less likely to produce extrapyramidal side-effects. The suggested doses are given in the table below. An attempt should be made to control the symptoms with the smallest possible dose, which should be tapered off at the earliest.

Medication	Starting dose (mg)	Maximum dose (mg)
Risperidone	0.5	2–3
Olanzapine	1–2.5	5–15
Quetiapine	12.5–25	100–200

Benzodiazepines form the first line of treatment for those suffering from delirium caused by alcohol withdrawal. Preparations with a short half-life are preferred in the elderly. Lorazepam (0.5–2 mg every 4 hours) can be given intravenously or intramuscularly until the behavioral problems are controlled. One may start reducing the dosage afterwards. One could reduce it by 50% daily while monitoring the symptoms and side-effects. However, benzodiazepines with a long half-life are best avoided. Even short-acting drugs can cause drowsiness and impair the person's attention and concentration. Vitamin supplements, especially thiamine and other B complex vitamins, are given to the patient routinely.

Non-pharmacological Management

It is necessary to educate the patient and caregivers about the condition. Providing reassurance, support, and explanations in simple terms should become a part of routine care. The caregivers and nursing staff should be informed about the transient brain dysfunction which is responsible for the symptoms of delirium.

The following interventions are known to help.

- Reorienting the patient frequently and scheduling his activities – the use of clocks, calendars, etc.
- Ensuring that the patient gets rest at night by avoiding the administration of injections/ medication during sleeping hours
- Reducing sensory deficits with the help of visual or hearing aids
- Avoiding physical restraints as much as possible, as it can cause adverse effects secondary to immobility and may result in injury
- Making attempts to accelerate mobilization and to ensure that the patient resumes his normal activities and social interaction as early as possible
- Minimizing changes in the staff and the patient's room
- Providing a quiet environment with a low level of lighting.

Prevention of Complications

Delirium is commonly associated with a number of complications. They should not be ignored and can be managed properly through good nursing care. The common complications are:

- Falls (common in hyperactive delirium)
- Pressure sores and deep vein thrombosis (common in hypoactive delirium)
- Urinary retention/incontinence
- Fecal impaction
- Dehydration.

BEHAVIORAL AND PSYCHOLOGICAL SYMPTOMS OF DEMENTIA

Behavioral and psychological symptoms of dementia (BPSD) is any behavior exhibited by a patient with dementia that is worrisome either for the patient, the caregiver or others. Some of the symptoms can be very disruptive and patients may be brought to the emergency services by their family members.

The common symptoms for which patients seek the help of emergency services are:

- Wandering in and out of the house
- Aggression – verbal, physical
- Agitation – pacing, anxiety
- Disinhibition – sexual disinhibition, removing clothes
- Vocalization – moaning, screaming
- Delusions and/or hallucinations.

MANAGEMENT OF BPSD

An accurate assessment of the underlying cause/s is the most important step. If there is evidence of superimposed delirium, then the delirium should be managed. If delirium is ruled out, one should consider other common factors known to cause/exacerbate BPSD. Factors such as pain, physical discomfort, wetness due to incontinence, hunger, and constipation can aggravate the symptoms. Since patients are often unable to talk accurately about their discomfort, it may remain unrecognized. Trying to find out whether these factors are present and relieving symptoms such as pain through the use of analgesics, etc. often helps. Symptoms such as aggression, agitation, delusional thinking, and hallucinations can be controlled by the short-term use of drugs.

Pharmacological Management

Antipsychotics are indicated for moderate to severe behavioral problems. These drugs need to be used with caution, especially because of concerns about their safety in patients with dementia (Ballard and Corbett 2010). One should start with low doses, increase the dose slowly and use the drug only for a short period. The dosages are indicated in the Annexure.

- Atypical antipsychotics such as risperidone, olanzapine, and quetiapine can be helpful in small doses.
- Avoid drugs with anticholinergic properties, such as chlorpromazine, trifluoperazine, and tricyclic antidepressants.
- Benzodiazepines have only a limited role to play as they are associated with recurrent falls, worsening of cognition and sometimes, paradoxical excitement.
- Antidepressants can be given for depression. Selective serotonin reuptake inhibitors (SSRIs) are preferred because of their safety and the lack of anticholinergic side-effects.

Caregiver Interventions

Educating the caregivers on BPSD could help them to cope with the patient's symptoms. Caregivers may be encouraged to use caregiver manuals/tips for care, etc., which they can obtain from websites or chapters of the Alzheimer's and Related Disorders Society of India (ARDSI) (http://www.alzheimer.org.in). An offer for support in case of future emergencies will always be appreciated. Caregivers may be informed about potential contact points which might come in handy in case of a future emergency.

PSYCHOSIS

Psychosis in late life may be due to the extension of symptoms of early-onset psychosis into late life or it may be a case of late-onset psychosis. Psychotic symptoms that appear for the first time in late life could be due to dementia or delirium. Sometimes, psychotic symptoms are the first sign of an underlying medical or neurological condition.

Psychotic symptoms may also be a manifestation of mood disorder, delusional disorder and late-onset schizophrenia. In depression, psychotic symptoms can be associated with severe agitation. Grandiose delusions and hallucinations are common in mania. Organic factors have to be ruled out in cases of late-onset psychosis as secondary mania is known to occur in this age group (Brooks and Hoblyn 2005).

Well-systematized, non-bizarre delusions in the absence of hallucinations and affective changes suggest delusional disorder. Late-onset schizophrenia is characterized by bizarre paranoid delusions and prominent hallucinations.

Worsening of psychotic symptoms or aggression associated with them, agitation, refusal of feeds, etc. can prompt people to seek an emergency consultation. The evaluation of the patient should include a detailed physical examination and investigations such as a complete blood count, an evaluation of the metabolic parameters and B12/folate levels, thyroid function tests, urine analysis, ECG, brain imaging studies (CT scan/ MRI scan) and VDRL.

Hospitalization is usually necessary for prompt control of the psychotic symptoms and to exclude organic causes. It can also help to relieve the stress of the caregivers. The main drugs used in the treatment of late-onset psychosis are antipsychotics. They should be given in the lowest effective doses. Patients with late-onset psychosis generally respond to doses that are 50%–70% of those needed to treat younger patients. The choice of the antipsychotic depends on the side-effect profile and the potential for drug interaction. Atypical antipsychotics are preferred in the elderly as they are less likely to produce extrapyramidal symptoms. The recommended dosages of some atypical antipsychotics are: risperidone 2–3 mg per day; olanzapine 5–15 mg per day; and quetiapine 100–200 mg per day. It is always better to initiate treatment with smaller doses and titrate the dose upwards while monitoring the effects on the target symptoms.

The psychosocial interventions that can be employed include the establishment of a good therapeutic relationship with the patient. This would improve the patient's adherence to medication and treatment plans. It is important to educate the caregivers and enable them to cope better with the symptoms of the illness.

DEPRESSION AND SUICIDAL BEHAVIOR

Depression is common in late life. Concurrent symptoms of comorbid physical illness and cognitive impairment can lead to the under-diagnosis of depression. Untreated depressive disorders associated with functional impairment (Gurland, Wilder and Berkman 1988) often lead to poor outcomes from medical illnesses such as ischemic heart disease and cerebrovascular disease. Patients usually visit the emergency room with problems such as suicidal behavior, refusal to eat, intense agitation, and severe fear and paranoia secondary to depression.

Among all the age groups, it is older adults who have the highest risk of death by suicide. Suicidal behavior is more planned and deliberate among the elderly than among others, and the means used are often lethal. Older people who have a history of suicidal ideation or who have earlier attempted suicide form a high-risk group. They need to be assessed for psychiatric morbidity and depression should be treated aggressively. Undetected, untreated depression is the most important cause of suicidal behavior in older people. Once the presence of depression has been identified, the condition should be explained to the patient and his caregivers and family members. The identification and adequate treatment of depression can indeed prevent a number of suicides among the elderly. The clinician should never dismiss depressive symptoms and suicidal behavior as insignificant in an older person.

The use of antidepressants can ameliorate depression. SSRIs are the preferred antidepressants for this age group. The dosage needed to treat depression in older people is by and large the same as that required by younger adults. It is important to prescribe an adequate dosage for the treatment of depression among the elderly.

Agitation is a state of restlessness. It is experienced by the patient as an inability to relax, while what the outsider observes is a state of restless activity. When the agitation is severe, the patient cannot sit for too long and usually paces up and down. Agitation is common among older patients with psychosis and depression. It can also occur among those with dementia and akathisia. The presence of agitation is a risk factor for suicide in persons with depression and psychotic disorders. Severe psychomotor agitation is often relieved by small doses of antipsychotics. One may choose to use very small doses of haloperidol (0.5–1.5 mg in divided doses) or olanzapine (2.5–5.0 mg in divided doses). Quetiapine is often preferred in the case of those with features of parkinsonism.

ANXIETY DISORDER

Anxiety disorders are less common in the later years of life than earlier on. However, if present, they can adversely affect the patient's quality of life. Among the anxiety disorders, it is panic disorders that can give rise to a psychiatric emergency. Panic attacks are characterized by intense anxiety, accompanied by multiple physical symptoms (autonomic arousal) and cognitive symptoms (fear of dying or going crazy). The intensity of the symptoms reaches a peak in 5–10 minutes and the attack lasts for 5–30 minutes. In the elderly, the symptoms might often suggest causes such as a "heart attack", and the fluctuating intensity of the symptoms may complicate the task of making a correct diagnosis.

SSRIs are the first line of treatment for anxiety disorders because their side-effect profile is more acceptable than that of other antidepressants such as tricyclic antidepressants. Benzodiazepines are best avoided because they can cause side-effects such as drowsiness and they increase the risk of falls. Short-acting benzodiazepines such as alprazolam (0.25–0.5 mg) can be used to relieve states of acute anxiety. However, this drug has a short half-life and thus needs to be used at least thrice a day. Prolonged use of benzodiazepines is associated with a risk of the development of dependence.

In most cases of psychiatric emergencies in the elderly, a thorough medical evaluation is warranted to identify the causes of the abnormal behavior. The pharmacological management of the patient should be tailor-made to meet the special needs of older people. Side-effects are a matter of great concern and one should always weigh the risks and benefits before initiating pharmacotherapy. The rates of suicide are high among this age group and a detailed psychiatric evaluation should be made if the patient has displayed suicidal behavior. Early identification and prompt management of depression can be life-saving.

REFERENCES

Ballard, C and Corbett, A 2010, Management of neuropsychiatric symptoms in people with dementia. *CNS Drugs,* 24, 729–739.

Brooks, JO III and Hoblyn, JC 2005, Secondary mania in older adults. *Am J Psychiatry,* 162, 2033–2038.

Gurland, BJ, Wilder, DE and Berkman, C 1988, Depression and disability in the elderly: Reciprocal relations and changes with age. *Int J Geriatr Psychiatry,* 3, 163–179.

Han, JH, Shintani, A, Eden, S, Morandi, A, Solberg, LM, Schnelle, J, Dittus, RS, Storrow, AB and Ely, EW 2010, Delirium in the emergency department: An independent predictor of death within 6 months. *Ann Emerg Med,* 56, 244-252.e1.

Heymann, A, Radtke, F, Schiemann, A, Lütz, A, MacGuill, M, Wernecke, KD and Spies, C 2010, Delayed treatment of delirium increases mortality rate in intensive care unit patients. *J Int Med Res,* 38, 1584–1595.

Khurana, V, Gambhir, IS and Kishore, D 2011, Evaluation of delirium in elderly: A hospital-based study. *Geriatr Gerontol Int,* 11, 467–473.

Leentjens, AF and van der Mast, RC 2005, Delirium in elderly people: An update. *Curr Opin Psychiatry,* 18, 325–330.

16 Psychiatric Emergencies after Terrorist Attacks

Murad Moosa Khan, Tania Nadeem, Nargis Asad

INTRODUCTION

Terrorist attacks and terrorism have become major global problems. Between 1961 and 2003 the US Department of State documented 228 acts of worldwide terrorism (DiMaggio and Galea 2006). Since 2003 there have been numerous terrorist attacks in more than 50 countries worldwide (Global Terrorism Index 2015). The single biggest terrorist attack has been the September 2001 (9/11) World Trade Center attacks in New York City in which almost 3000 people were killed.

Since 9/11 other terrorist attacks such as the Bali (Indonesia) nightclub bombing in October 2002, the Madrid (Spain) train bombings in March 2004, the London (UK) bombings in July 2005, the Mumbai (India) attack in 2008, the Oslo and Utoya (Norway) attacks in July 2011, the Army Public School, Peshawar (Pakistan) attack in December 2014 and the Brussels (Belgium) attacks in March 2016 have highlighted the global threat of terrorism and the fact that virtually no country is safe from such attacks.

It is interesting to note the pattern of pre- and post-9/11 terror attacks. Terrorism pre-9/11 was concentrated in Latin America and Asia, but shifted to the Middle East post-9/11 – and countries such as Peru, Chile, and El Salvador completely disappear from the top 10 most affected countries. More than a quarter of all terrorist attacks between 9/11 and 2008 took place in Iraq (Nagdy and Roser 2015).

Apart from the above-mentioned incidents that gained massive media coverage, there have been scores of terror attacks in countries as diverse as Iraq, Syria, Egypt, Yemen, Afghanistan, Pakistan, Turkey, Nigeria, Kenya, Somalia, Russia, Israel, Thailand, Philippines, Sri Lanka, Northern Ireland, France, Australia, and India, among many others, resulting in thousands of casualties. Many of these attacks have been suicide bombings. The number of countries experiencing more than 50 deaths rose to 24 in 2013; the previous high had been 19 in 2008 (Global Terrorism Index 2015). Eighty percent of lives lost to terrorism in 2013 were in only five countries: Iraq, Afghanistan, Pakistan, Nigeria, and Syria. Since 2000, only about 5% of all the estimated 107,000 terrorism-related deaths have occurred in developed countries, members of the Organization for Economic Co-operation and Development, which includes most of Europe and the USA (Global Terrorism Index 2015).

Terrorist attacks can be considered as a form of interpersonal violence (Fischer and Ai 2008). However, classification of terror attacks can be difficult as different groups have different interpretations of what constitutes a terror attack, depending on the circumstances and who the attack is carried out against. Notwithstanding the academic classifications, all terror attacks appear to share a number of commonalities: terror attacks target innocent civilians with the aim of spreading terror and fear among the general population; the attacks attract huge media coverage and in this age of instant communication, terrorists can get their agenda across almost instantly; terror attacks may be politically, economically, ideologically, culturally, or religiously motivated and any country can be a victim (Fischer and Ai 2008).

As a result of the increased incidence of the phenomena, there has been an increase in research interest as well, in particular on the mental health consequences of terror attacks.

MENTAL HEALTH NEEDS AFTER A TERROR ATTACK

The assessment of mental health needs of survivors following a terror attack is often overlooked, because unlike physical injuries in such incidents, psychological wounds are not so apparent (North and Pfefferbaum 2013). However, accurate assessment of mental health issues and needs is vital, both for effective emergency response as well as to prevent long-term psychological morbidity. Several studies highlight short-term and long-term threat to mental health, both directly from being a victim of terror attacks but also indirectly from seeing images or hearing and reading about the incident.

Although most studies focus on negative impacts on mental health, such as emotional stress and post-traumatic stress disorders (PTSD), studies also highlight the potential positive outcomes on the resilience side such as the concept of post-traumatic growth (PTG).

RAPID RESPONSE AFTER A TERRORIST ATTACK

Following a terrorist attack it is critical to attend to the survivors' physical and medical needs as quickly and as efficiently as possible to prevent loss of life and reduce injuries. These should take precedence over any psychological concerns. Ideally, emergency response should come from law enforcement agencies, rescue services, ambulance services, fire fighters, and emergency medical teams, all working in tandem with each other. This may happen in countries that are well prepared for such situations. However, most low- and middle-income countries (LMICs) lack the necessary infrastructure or resources to cope with a sudden attack with a large number of casualties. A disorganized response can add to the chaos and distress, rather than relief for the survivors (Tucker and Ng 2004).

As seen after multiple terror attacks and suicide bombings in Pakistan and elsewhere in LMICs, extreme chaos initially stems from people trying to locate their family members. In 2013 two apartment complexes in a town in Karachi, Pakistan, were targeted with high explosive bombs that left many families homeless. The lack of coordinated response from different agencies added to the chaos and confusion. It is vital to provide easy access to lists of the dead and injured and their locations, as soon as possible. Well-structured methods of information sharing and communication and safety and accommodation for the survivors should be provided. Institutional and social support is well documented as important predictors of recovery from traumatic stress reactions (Thabet and Vostanis 1999).

PSYCHOLOGICAL REACTIONS

Terrorism creates immense mental suffering due to exposure to violence, fear of death, and feelings of lack of control (Leon and Polusny 2004). In the acute phase, survivors may experience a range of emotional reactions including: symptoms of acute stress, anxiety, extreme distress, shock, numbness, disbelief, physical symptoms such as loss of appetite, sleep disturbance, aches and pains, fearfulness about self and others, and depression.

It is important to recognize that many of these responses are normal reactions to highly unusual and abnormal events, and for most individuals, the reactions will diminish and settle down with time. Hence, reassurance and helping survivors use their natural coping mechanisms, along with some social support may be sufficient. For most people recovery is spontaneous and they are able to return to normal daily living. The existing research indicates that over time, most of those exposed to trauma recover without formal psychological interventions (Leon and Polusny 2004).

Loss

Dealing with loss is a major component of helping people after terrorist attacks. In such incidents, death is sudden, survivors may have serious injuries, and hospital staff may be overwhelmed due to the sheer numbers of injured people who may require help (McLauchlan 1990). Healthy family members may need help in disclosing information about a loved one who has died to an injured surviving family member. Families feel unsure about disclosing the information and want to know when to tell and how to tell. The principles of breaking bad news are useful to follow in such situations (McLauchlan 1990). Generally, supporting families and encouraging them to communicate honestly is important.

With children, who may have lost parents, this can become even more complicated depending on the child's developmental age (Leon and Polusny 2004). Children under 8 years of age cannot understand the irreversibility of death and might recurrently expect their parents to return. Thus, this conversation might have to be repeated multiple times with a child.

Acute Stress Disorder

Acute stress disorder can occur after being exposed to a traumatic, life-threatening event and results in many dissociative symptoms along with feelings of detachment and amnesia. It also includes hyperarousal, avoidance, and re-living of symptoms (Creamer *et al.* 2004). These symptoms may last up to one month after the trauma. Following the terrorist attack in Mumbai, India in 2008, 30% of the 70 victims treated at a public hospital were diagnosed with acute stress disorder (Balasinorwala and Shah 2010). Acute stress disorder does not indicate that the person will develop PTSD. However, hyperarousal and symptoms of re-experiencing trauma are better predictors of an ultimate diagnosis of PTSD (Creamer *et al.* 2004).

Post-traumatic Stress Disorder (PTSD)

The most commonly reported diagnosis after a traumatic event, such as a terrorist attack, is PTSD, followed by depression, anxiety disorders, and substance abuse (Sareen 2014). There is also high comorbidity between these disorders.

Prevalence figures for PTSD are as varied as the cultures where such studies have been conducted. A multi-ethnic study employing nationals from Saudi Arabia, Turkey, and Iran who had immigrated to Sweden reported diverse PTSD figures, with highest prevalence in Iranians at 69%, followed by 59% and 53% in Saudis and Turks, respectively, whereas only 29% of the Swedes reported similar symptoms, all having been exposed to previous traumatic events (Al-Saffar *et al.* 2003).

There is appreciable variability in reported occurrence of PTSD after natural versus man-made disasters such as war or terrorist attacks, ranging between 1.5% and 67% after natural disasters and as high as 99% after man-made disasters (Wang *et al.* 2011).

Lifetime rates of PTSD vary according to the location of the study and type of study population, ranging from 1% to 40% (Wang *et al.* 2011). A terrorist attack, due to its objective of terrorizing people, leads to an increase in symptoms of PTSD in the general population. Many individuals' symptoms recede with time and only a few are left who need professional help. As seen after the September 11 attacks in New York, rates of PTSD increased to 11%–13%, but decreased to less than 3% in 2 months after the attack (Whalley and Brewin 2007).

Sub-threshold PTSD can also be functionally impairing. About 5.3% of New York residents showed such symptoms 6 months after the September 11 attacks, which detrimentally affected the quality of their lives (Sareen 2014).

Individuals who are at risk of developing longer-term psychiatric pathology need to be identified early. Individual risk factors include: female gender, lower intellect, previous exposure to trauma, family history or personal prior history of psychiatric illness, personality disorder (borderline and antisocial), poor social support, and poor coping skills (Sareen 2014). The severity of trauma, personal physical injury, loss of family members, head injuries, or limb amputations can increase chances of severe reaction to stress. Post-trauma, poor social and financial support, admission to intensive care unit (ICU), increased pain and heart rate and dissociative symptoms also increase chances of pathology after attacks (Sareen 2014). Such individuals need to be monitored more closely after trauma to treat pathology as soon as it arises.

Wilcox *et al.* (2009) have shown that high rates of suicidality are associated with PTSD. PTSD leads to long-term morbidity due to interpersonal relationship problems, parenting problems, increased anger, increased alcohol use, and occupational problems. It is also associated with an increased rate of medical problems such as cardiovascular issues, respiratory disease, metabolic problems, neurological issues, and joint and bone problems (Wilcox, Storr and Breslau 2009).

SPECIAL GROUPS

Two groups need special mention: the first-responders and children. The former include police officers, fire fighters, or ambulance service personnel. In terror attacks the first responders face large-scale traumatic events and can be affected emotionally by what they witness. Prevalence estimates of PTSD in first responders range from 6% to more than 20% in different studies and have been found to be related to more suicidal ideation, reduced quality of life, poor physical health, more medical visits (Sterud, Ekeberg and Hem 2006; Berger *et al.* 2007).

A study carried out on Pakistan emergency responders (*n*=125) showed that 15% of participants exposed to terrorist attacks reported clinically significant levels of PTSD symptoms and between 11% and 16% reported heightened levels of anxiety, depression, and/or somatic symptoms (Razik, Ehring and Emmelkamp 2013). Neither the experience of terrorist attacks per se nor the severity of the attack experienced was related to symptom severities.

Children and adolescents are another group that requires special attention. There is much less information about the impact of terror attacks, as well as the effectiveness of treatment approaches on children and adolescents (Leon and Polusny 2004). In some of the recent incidents such as the attack in Beslan, Russia and on the Army Public School in Peshawar, Pakistan, children were specifically targeted by terrorists. Children and adolescents respond differently to acts of terrorism than adults. This may be related more to their developmental level of cognitive and emotional functioning. Children's response to traumatic events may manifest itself more in terms of school performance and behaviors rather than emotional reactions (Leon and Polusny 2004). This is often overlooked.

TRAUMATIC STRESS REACTIONS FROM AN ETHNO-CULTURAL PERSPECTIVE

Psychiatric emergencies following trauma from terrorism are universal. However, manifestations at individual and community level vary across different cultures. Culture shapes the psychological manifestations of terrorism-related emergencies. Due to threats to security escalate on the international front, there is increased need for understanding the cultural context where the trauma happens, to better inform management practices in a contextually relevant manner.

Differences in the nature of traumatic stress symptoms have been linked to individualistic and collectivistic cultural differences (Elsass 2001). Cultures also vary in extent to which expression of psychological distress is considered acceptable, e.g. Chinese are generally reluctant to disclose and express distress and attribute reasons of distress to external and physical reasons (Al-Saffar *et al.* 2003). Bhutanese refugees attribute distress to angered gods, dissatisfied spirits, and witchcraft (Shrestha *et al.* 1998). Survivors of the 2005 Pakistan earthquake attributed the disaster to being "punished by God for our sins and lack of spirituality" (Feder *et al.* 2013).

Palestinian youth reported frequent conversion symptoms, behavioral problems, and psychosomatic complaints in response to traumatic experiences (Punamäki *et al.*

2005). "Weak heart syndrome" is reported among Khmer refugees closely resembling PTSD and panic disorder (Marsella and Christopher 2004).

Understanding individual and collective response to trauma in different cultures (and sub-cultures) is important as many times the international response to disaster situations means that medical and mental health professionals may come from different countries and cultures.

TELEVISED TRAUMA AND MENTAL HEALTH

In today's highly interconnected and globalized world, mass media – satellite television, social, and print media, turn local incidents into national and global events by transmitting the negative impact of disasters to people far beyond those directly exposed (Silver *et al.* 2013). Media coverage of major terrorist events tends to be graphic and intense, with images of death and destruction, chaos, and suffering of the victims.

Research has shown that repeated viewing of such images can be traumatizing for some individuals and may affect both their physical and mental health (even among those indirectly exposed) and causing long-term psychopathology (Silver *et al.* 2013).

There is now good research evidence to suggest that caution should be used in the kind of images that should be shown and guidelines should be developed so that a balance could be maintained between accurate news reporting and the potentially harmful effects of such reporting. PTSD and depression are serious mental conditions and can cause impairment and disability. It is therefore imperative that every effort should be made to prevent their occurrence or exacerbation of symptoms following a traumatic event.

ASSESSMENT OF PSYCHIATRIC EMERGENCIES

Post-terror attack assessments need to be carried out at both community-level as well as individual-level (Ruzek *et al.* 2004). The former is required to allocate resources, inform planning and delivery of services as well as carrying out interventions, while the latter requires clinical evaluation, diagnosis, and appropriate referral (Nucifora *et al.* 2011). For both types of assessments, resources – human as well as material, are required, particularly if sample populations to be assessed are large (North and Pfefferbaum 2013). Use of screening instruments in such situations is valuable. However, such screening instruments need to be simple and brief, culturally and linguistically reliable and valid, and should be easy to administer and score (Brewin 2005).

For community-level assessment, information about prevalence and risk factors for mental disorders, and resources and services available in a particular community before a disaster, are important so that post-disaster response can be planned accordingly (North and Pfefferbaum 2013). This information is not always available, particularly in LMICs.

Individual assessments are critical and can identify any pre-existing psychiatric disorders, level of functioning, attitudes and beliefs, and symptoms such as insomnia or hypervigilance. Those individuals identified as having psychiatric disorders would require referral to formal psychiatric services to be assessed for the most appropriate intervention (North and Pfefferbaum 2013). In addition, acute crisis situations, such as active suicidal ideation, acute psychosis, or panic states may require referral to psychiatric services. Pre-existing psychiatric disorders, both diagnosed as well as undiagnosed, are frequently unearthed following a disaster situation and require stabilization.

In many instances, the previous treatment individuals were on may get disrupted and would need to be re-established as early as possible. In other situations, a previously stable individual may decompensate as a result of the incident. In both the Hurricane Katrina and Oklahoma City bombing, 40% and 63% of survivors seen in mental health clinic had a pre-existing psychiatric disorder (North *et al.* 1999).

Assessment of psychiatric emergencies should also include factors related to physical safety, medical conditions, housing, food, family, and psychological support (Silove 2013). For children and adolescents, this should include restoration of school and social/peer-related activities.

Diagnosis of PTSD is based on a clinical interview and assessment. Detailed history including social functioning prior to trauma, social support systems, coping skills, and sleeps problems, all should be assessed thoroughly. Suicide risk assessment is essential (Sareen 2014).

In addition to comorbid medical conditions, food, and shelter, assessment in adults will also require an assessment of their income-generation activities. Geriatric populations in particular need close monitoring of physical and neuropsychiatric conditions, as well as mobility issues.

MANAGEMENT

Although most people who are exposed to terror attacks, either directly or indirectly, will not develop psychiatric disorders, almost all people so exposed will experience some degree of distress, even for a brief period of time. The principles of management of psychiatric reactions after a terrorist act are guided by the principles of management of trauma following any other acute disaster. In all such situations the underlying objective is to provide early psychosocial support and prevent psychological morbidity in the medium to long term.

It is useful for all health workers, who deal with psychiatric reactions following a terrorist attack, to have a conceptual framework in order to improve the delivery of services for persons in a traumatic state. Roberts (2002) suggests a three-part conceptual framework that may be helpful in serving as a foundation model to initiate, implement, and evaluate a coordinated crisis intervention and trauma treatment program. The three parts determine sequentially which assessment and intervention strategies to use first, second, and third.

It is imperative for all emergency services professionals to be trained so that they can respond immediately and effectively to traumatic events. The training should include being able to differentiate between acute stress, normal grief, acute crisis episodes, trauma reactions, and PTSD (Roberts 2002).

In the immediate aftermath of a terrorist attack, a full assessment of the situation and individual must take place. Early contact with the survivors reduces the risk of acute stress reactions becoming chronic stress disorders. Lerner and Shelton (2001) provide a useful guide for Acute Traumatic Stress Management (ATSM), the first three steps of which are: (i) Assess for danger/safety for self and others; (ii) Consider the type and extent of property damage and/or physical injury and the way the injury was sustained (e.g. from an explosion); and (iii) Evaluate the level of responsiveness – is the individual alert, in pain, aware of what has occurred, on in emotional shock or under the influence of drugs.

Roberts (2002) also provides a useful framework to measure the personal impact in the immediate aftermath of potentially stressful and crisis-producing events. The framework includes the following:

1. Spatial dimensions, i.e. the closer the survivor is to the center of event, the greater the stress. Similarly, the closer the person's relationship to the dead victim, the greater the likelihood of entering into a crisis state.
2. Subjective time clock, i.e. the greater the duration of the exposure to the trauma and exposure to sensory experiences, e.g. odor of gasoline or smell of fire, the greater the stress.
3. Re-occurrence, i.e. the more perceived likelihood that the trauma will happen again, the greater the likelihood of intense fears, which contribute to an active crisis state in the survivor.

MENTAL HEALTH INTERVENTIONS FOLLOWING A TERROR ATTACK

There are many models of mental health interventions for psychiatric emergencies following a disaster including terror attacks. Almost all address the same basic issues, i.e. to provide support for psychological distress while the person adapts to the changed situation. North and Pfefferbaum (2013) provide an excellent overview of common early psychosocial interventions after trauma. The three best-known interventions are psychological first aid, psychological debriefing, and crisis counseling. These are summarized below.

Psychological First Aid

The principles of psychological first aid (PFA) are similar to physical first aid. PFA is an example of early mental health intervention and aims to stabilize the survivor of a disaster situation by meeting the immediate physical needs such as safety, security, and physical injuries, followed by emotional/psychological needs (Reyes and Elhai 2004). The basic premise is to help the victim tide over the initial shock of the attack by attending to the psychological distress. Ideally, all emergency aid providers and emergency health workers should be trained in PFA, which can be delivered in diverse settings (Young 2006). One of the biggest advantages of PFA is that, like physical first aid, non-clinicians can also be trained in providing it (Reyes and Elhai 2004).

Psychological Debriefing

Psychological debriefing, including Critical Incident Stress Management (CISM), is another type of mental health intervention that is provided hours or days post-trauma. The main elements of psychological debriefing are "emotional ventilation, trauma processing and psychoeducation" (North and Pfefferbaum 2013). There is some controversy about its effectiveness, particularly in PTSD and those at risk for PTSD may worsen with debriefing. Psychological debriefing was actually intended to normalize survivors' reactions, process their trauma experiences, address psychological distress, and enhance resilience (North and Pfefferbaum 2013). It was not intended to prevent or treat individuals with PTSD, who should be referred to psychiatric services instead.

Crisis Counseling

Crisis counseling is another form of intervention that can be delivered by trained crisis workers in acute disaster settings (Reyes and Elhai 2004). It has many elements similar to psychological first aid and can be delivered to individuals as well as groups to help survivors understand their reactions, enhance coping, consider options, and connect with other services. Like the other interventions in acute disaster settings, crisis counseling is not a substitute for those individuals who otherwise require more formal psychiatric assessment and care (Norris and Rosen 2009).

In addition to the specific interventions described above, some general measure can also help mitigate the effect of the trauma. These include: mobilizing community and religious resources along with family and other social support; providing factual information to victims and larger population; disseminating information about common psychological symptoms and how to manage them, following a terror incident utilizing print, social, and broadcast media: educating teachers in enabling children to deal with the trauma; and preventing mass distress by responsible media reporting (US Department of Health and Human Services 2005).

Other useful measures include encouraging people to exercise, having meals with family members, restore normal routine including sending children to school, going to work, paying attention to sleep, and having a healthy diet (US Department of Health and Human Services 2005).

The underlying principle should be to individualizing help according to the person's need, temperament, and social support.

Pharmacotherapy

Pharmacotherapy can be useful for psychiatric disorders related to trauma including those following a terror attack. In early period following a trauma, medications for sleep and excessive anxiety may be required (North *et al.* 2008). Later, medications may be required for symptoms of PTSD or major clinical depression. Selective serotonin reuptake inhibitors (SSRIs) (fluoxetine, sertraline, and paroxetine) and SNRIs (venlafaxine) help with all groups of symptoms of PTSD, anxiety, and depression. The fact that there is high degree of comorbidity of PTSD and major depression makes the use of antidepressants particularly useful. Evidence also suggests that extended use of SSRIs, beyond the acute phase, can further improve symptoms and prevent relapse (Ravindran and Stein 2009). Their limitation is the delayed onset of improvement. Benzodiazepines (clonazepam, alprazolam, and temazepam) can be helpful as adjunctive medications for individuals with sleep disturbance, irritability, anxiety, and other hyperarousal symptoms. Trazadone and zopiclone can also be used for individuals with sleep problems. Centrally acting alpha-2 adrenergic agonists, such as clonidine, and alpha-1 adrenergic blockers, such as prazosin, are useful for insomnia, nightmares, flashbacks, hypervigilance, and agitation (Ravindran and Stein 2009). There is some evidence of the efficacy of atypical antipsychotics (olanzapine and risperidone) as adjunctive treatment in individuals with agitation, severe flashbacks, and anxiety (Sareen 2014).

Victims whose psychiatric medications may have been interrupted due to the disaster must have their medications restored as early as possible.

Post-traumatic Growth (PTG)

Despite extreme psychological distress that individuals may experience following a major trauma like a terrorist attack, it has been seen that with proper support there can also be "post-traumatic growth" (PTG), defined as "the experience of positive change that occurs as a result of the struggle with highly challenging life crises" (Ravindran and Stein 2009). These positive changes may include the development of new perspectives and personal growth (Knudsen *et al.* 2005).

In the struggle to cope with the trauma, individuals may develop "alternative interpretations of the crisis, perceived benefits or new meaning and purposes of life" (Tedeschi and Calhoun 2004). Over time, this positive outlook may counter the negative effects of the trauma and lead to psychological well-being.

Research has shown that PTG is generally characterized by three major aspects: (i) more meaningful interpersonal relationships; (ii) new views of the self; and (iii) changed worldviews (including changed political views) (Ai *et al.* 2006). Also, individuals value life more and there is more appreciation of good health.

However, it is important to note that the concept of PTG is a relatively new one and it is still evolving. Preliminary research findings also suggest that personality styles, coping mechanisms, and resiliency factors may play a much greater role in how victims react to trauma (King and Hicks 2009). More research is needed in this area to clarify the concept. Nevertheless, there are important clinical implications of PTG, and mental health professionals need to be aware of the factors that can contribute of PTG in victims. As more research evidence on PTG accumulates, it may be possible in the future to design therapeutic interventions incorporating PTG that are evidence-based and empirically tested, which promote positive changes as part of the recovery process from trauma (Dekel, Mandl and Solomon 2011).

SUMMARY AND FUTURE DIRECTIONS

Terrorism and terror attacks have become modern-day realities and are major global concerns. Although it is a form of interpersonal violence, by its very nature it has the potential to affect a huge number of people, both directly and indirectly. Research has revealed the mental health consequences of terrorism that, if not properly addressed, can cause short-term and long-term morbidity. It is, therefore, important to study the impact of terrorism on mental health.

Most research on mental health consequences of terrorism has been conducted in the USA, particularly following the 9/11 terrorist attacks, with little evidence from Europe, Middle East, Africa, or Asia, though these regions of the world are as affected (if not more) by terrorism. Hence, it is imperative that future research should focus on these areas of the world as well, to contextualize the social, cultural, and religious effects of terrorism and how these factors moderate the mental health responses to such acts. It is possible that people in different countries and regions of the world view terrorism differently, and use different coping strategies. For example, people in one region or country may use religion as an important coping strategy than in other countries or the political context of terrorism in some regions may evoke an entirely different community and/or individual response, which moderates the mental health response.

Future research must address some of the social and economic effects of terrorism. After the December 2014 terror attack on the school in Peshawar, Pakistan, the government directed all schools in the country to beef up their security, the costs of which were substantial and were passed on to the students.

The long-term mental health consequences of terrorism are largely unknown. There is a need for longitudinal studies to build the evidence base and to inform policy and develop services. LMICs in particular should consider each terror incident as an opportunity to advocate for mental health services and programs. In Pakistan, for example, in the aftermath of the December 2014 school attack, the government made plans to set up the National Action Plan for Mental Health and Psychosocial Support (NAP-MHPSS) to address the mental health consequences of disasters and terror attacks, though little progress has been made since then (*The Express Tribune* 2014).

There is also need for research in the area of positive aspects of terror attacks such as PTG, protective factors, and resiliency factors. Very few studies have been conducted on the positive effects of terrorism on community (as opposed to individual) mental health based on factors such as cohesion, unity, and interfaith understanding.

Despite the growth in terrorism worldwide, very few countries have invested in dealing with the mental health consequences of terrorism, and overall this remains a neglected area. This is of particular concern for LMICs of South Asia, Africa, and Middle East, many of which have become targets for terror attacks. Countries in these regions lack resources, but more importantly, mental health services are poorly developed in these countries. For example, in some regions most affected by terrorism the psychiatrist–population ratio is one psychiatrist to a million people (Fricchione *et al.* 2012). In the event of a large terrorist attack, health services, including mental health services, are quickly overwhelmed. Hence, in addition to improving mental health services in these settings, training non-mental health professionals in basic counseling skills and psychological first aid may be a way of addressing the problem. All emergency health staff, first responders, paraprofessionals, and teachers should be included in this exercise.

CONCLUSION

Terror attacks and terrorism will, unfortunately, continue to remain serious challenges of the modern world for the foreseeable future. The health and mental health consequences of such incidents will continue to challenge the global health community. Meeting this challenge requires a concerted and collaborative approach at international, regional, national, as well as local level. By doing so, short- and long-term mental health consequences of such acts on individuals and communities could be addressed effectively.

REFERENCES

Ai, AL, Evans-Campbell, T, Santangelo, LK and Cascio, T 2006, The traumatic impact of the September 11, 2001, terrorist attacks and the potential protection of optimism. *J Interpers Violence,* 21, 689–700.

Al-Saffar, S, Borgå, P, Edman, G and Hällström, T 2003, The aetiology of posttraumatic stress disorder in four ethnic groups in outpatient psychiatry. *Soc Psychiatry Psychiatr Epidemiol,* 38, 456–462.

Balasinorwala, VP and Shah, N 2010, Acute stress disorder in hospitalised victims of 26/11 – terror attack on Mumbai, India. *J Indian Med Assoc,* 108, 757; 759–760.

Berger, W, Figueira, I, Maurat, AM, Bucassio, EP, Vieira, I, Jardim, SR, Coutinho, ES, Mari, JJ and Mendlowicz, MV 2007, Partial and full PTSD in Brazilian ambulance workers: Prevalence and impact on health and on quality of life. *J Trauma Stress,* 20, 637–642.

Brewin, CR 2005, Systematic review of screening instruments for adults at risk of PTSD. *J Trauma Stress* 18, 53–62.

Creamer, M, O'Donnell, ML and Pattison, P 2004, Acute stress disorder is of limited benefit in predicting post-traumatic stress disorder in people surviving traumatic injury. *Behav Res Ther,* 42, 315–328.

Dekel, S, Mandl, C and Solomon, Z 2011, Shared and predictors of posttraumatic growth and distress. *J Clin Psychol,* 67, 241–252.

DiMaggio, C and Galea, S 2006, The behavioral consequences of terrorism: A meta-analysis. *Acad Emerg Med,* 13, 559–566.

Elsass, P 2001, Individual and collective traumatic memories: A qualitative study of post-traumatic stress disorder symptoms in two Latin American localities. *Transcult Psychiatry,* 38, 306–316.

Feder, A, Ahmad, S, Lee, EJ, Morgan, JE, Singh, R, Smith, BW, Southwick, SM and Charney, DS 2013, Coping and PTSD symptoms in Pakistani earthquake survivors: Purpose in life, religious coping and social support. *J Affect Disord,* 147, 156–163.

Fischer, P and Ai, AL 2008, International terrorism and mental health: Recent research and future directions, *J Interpers Violence,* 23, 339–361.

Fricchione, GL, Borba, CP, Alem, A, Shibre, T, Carney, JR and Henderson, DC 2012, Capacity building in global mental health: Professional training. *Harv Rev Psychiatry*, 20, 47–57.

Global Terrorism Index 2015. Available at http://www.visionofhumanity.org/#/page/our-gti-findings.

King, L and Hicks, J 2009, Detecting and constructing meaning in life events. *J Positive Psychology,* 4, 317–330.

Knudsen, HK, Roman, PM, Johnson, JA and Ducharme, LJ 2005, A changed America? The effects of September 11th on depressive symptoms and alcohol consumption. *J Health Soc Behav,* 46, 260–273.

Leon, G and Polusny, MA 2004, Introduction to the special theme issue on psychosocial issues in disasters and terrorism. *Prehospital Disaster Med,* 19, 2–3.

Lerner, MD and Shelton, R 2001, Acute traumatic stress management, ATSM: Addressing emergent psychological needs during traumatic events. American Academy of Experts in Traumatic Stress.

Marsella, AJ and Christopher, MA 2004, Ethnocultural considerations in disasters: An overview of research, issues, and directions. *Psychiatric Clinics of North America,* 27, 521–539.

McLauchlan, CA 1990, ABC of major trauma. Handling distressed relatives and breaking bad news. *BMJ,* 301, 1145–1149.

Nagdy, M and Roser M 2015, "Terrorism". Published online at OurWorldInData.org. Available at http://ourworldindata.org/data/war-peace/terrorism/ [Online Resource].

Norris, FH and Rosen, CS 2009, Innovations in disaster mental health services and evaluation: National, state, and local responses to Hurricane Katrina (introduction to the special issue). *Adm Policy Ment Health,* 36, 159–164.

North, C, King, R, Fowler, R, Polatin, P, Smith, R, LaGrone, H, Tyler, D, Larkin, G and Pepe, P 2008, Psychiatric disorders among transported hurricane evacuees: Acute-phase findings in a large receiving shelter site. *Psychiatr Ann,* 38, 104–113.

North, CS, Nixon, SJ, Shariat, S, Mallonee, S, McMillen, JC, Spitznagel, EL and Smith, EM 1999, Psychiatric disorders among survivors of the Oklahoma City bombing. *JAMA,* 282, 755–762.

North, CS and Pfefferbaum, B 2013, Mental health response to community disasters: A systematic review. *JAMA,* 310, 507–518. doi:10.1001/jama.2013.107799

North, CS 2013, Rethinking disaster mental health response in a post-9/11 world. *Can J Psychiatry,* 58, 125–127.

Nucifora, FC, Jr, Hall, RC and Everly, GS Jr 2011, Reexamining the role of the traumatic stressor and the trajectory of posttraumatic distress in the wake of disaster. *Disaster Med Public Health Prep,* 5 (Suppl 2), S172–S175.

Punamäki, RL, Komproe, IH, Qouta, S, Elmasri, M and de Jong JT 2005, The role of peritraumatic dissociation and gender in the association between trauma and mental health in a Palestinian community sample. *Am J Psychiatry,* 162, 545–551.

Ravindran, LN and Stein, MB 2009, Pharmacotherapy of PTSD: Premises, principles, and priorities. *Brain Res,* 1293, 24–39.

Razik, S, Ehring, T and Emmelkamp, PMG 2013, Psychological consequences of terrorist attacks: Prevalence and predictors of mental health problems in Pakistani emergency responders. *Psychiatry Res,* 207, 80–85.

Reyes, G and Elhai, JD 2004, Psychosocial interventions in the early phases of disasters. *Psychother Theory Res Prac Train,* 41, 399–411.

Roberts, AR 2002, Assessment, crisis intervention and trauma treatment: The integrative ACT intervention model. *Brief Treat Crisis Interv,* 2, 1–21.

Ruzek, JI, Young, BH, Cordova, MJ and Flynn, BW 2004, Integration of disaster mental health services with emergency medicine. *Prehosp Disaster Med,* 19, 46–53.

Sareen, J 2014, Posttraumatic stress disorder in adults: Impact, comorbidity, risk factors, and treatment. *Can J Psychiatry*, 59, 460–467.

Shrestha, NM, Sharma, B, Van Ommeren, M, Regmi, S, Makaju, R, Komproe, I, Shrestha, GB and de Jong, JT 1998, Impact of torture on refugees displaced within the developing world: Symptomatology among Bhutanese refugees in Nepal. *JAMA*, 280, 443–448.

Silove, D 2013, The ADAPT model: A conceptual framework for mental health and psychosocial programming in post conflict settings. *Intervention,* 11, 237–248.

Silver, RC, Holman, EA, Andersen, JP, Poulin, M, McIntosh, DN and Gil-Rivas V 2013, Mental- and physical-health effects of acute exposure to media images of the September 11, 2001, attacks and the Iraq War. *Psychol Sci*, 24, 1623–1634.

Sterud, T, Ekeberg, O and Hem E. 2006, Health status in the ambulance services: A systematic review. *BMC Health Serv Res*, 6, 82.

Tedeschi, R and Calhoun, L 2004, Posttraumatic growth: Conceptual foundations and empirical evidence. *Psychol Inq* 15, 1–18.

Thabet, AAM and Vostanis, P 1999, Post-traumatic stress reactions in children of war. *J Child Psychol Psychiatry*, 40, 385–391.

The Express Tribune, December 30, 2014. *Battling PTSD: Psychological Trauma Centres to be set up*. Available at http://tribune.com.pk/story/814254/battling-ptsd-psychological-trauma-centres-to-be-set-up/

Tucker, P and Ng, AT 2004, Helping adults after disaster strikes. *Disaster psychiatry handbook*, pp. 20–27.

U.S. Department of Health and Human Services 2005. DHHS Pub. No. SMA 4025. Rockville, MD: Center for Mental Health Services, Substance Abuse and Mental Health Services Administration, 2005; 2005. Mental health response to mass violence and terrorism: A field guide.

Wang, L, Zhang, J, Shi, Z, Zhou, M, Li, Z, Zhang, K, Liu, Z and Elhai, JD 2011, Comparing alternative factor models of PTSD symptoms across earthquake victims and violent riot witnesses in China: Evidence for a five-factor model. *J Anxiety Disord*, 25, 771–776.

Whalley, MG and Brewin, CR 2007, Mental health following terrorist attacks. *Br J Psychiatry*, 190, 94–96.

Wilcox, HC, Storr, CL and Breslau, N 2009, Posttraumatic stress disorder and suicide attempts in a community sample of urban American young adults. *Arch Gen Psychiatry*, 66, 305–311.

Young, BH 2006, The immediate response to disaster: Guidelines for adult psychological first aid. In: Ritchie, EC, Watson, PJ and Friedman, MJ (eds). *Interventions following mass violence and disasters: Strategies for mental health practice*, pp. 135–154. New York: Guilford Press.

Annexure: Suggested Dosages

Drugs for psychosis	Dosage	Side-effects
Risperidone	2–3 mg per day Start with lower doses (0.5 mg)	Parkinsonism, weight gain, Tardive dyskinesia
Olanzapine	5–15 mg per day in divided doses Start with lower doses (2.5 mg)	Sedation, Parkinsonism, weight gain, Tardive dyskinesia
Quetiapine	100–200 in divided doses Start with lower doses (25 mg)	Sedation

Drugs for depression	Dosage	Side-effects
Sertraline	50–100 mg per day Start with lower doses (25 mg)	Insomnia, headache, hyponatremia
Escitalopram	10–20 mg per day Start with lower doses (5 mg)	Insomnia, headache, hyponatremia

Drugs for anxiety	Dosage	Side-effects
Sertraline	50–100 mg per day Start with lower doses (25 mg)	Insomnia, headache, hyponatremia
Escitalopram	10–20 mg per day Start with lower doses (5 mg)	Insomnia, headache, hyponatremia
Alprazolam	0.25–0.5 mg per day	Drowsiness

Short-term use of drugs for agitation associated with depression	Dosage	Side-effects
Haloperidol	0.5–1.5 mg per day in divided doses	Parkinsonism
Olanzapine	2.5–5 mg per day in divided doses	Sedation, parkinsonism
Quetiapine	25–50 mg per day in divided doses	Sedation

Index

* In this index, the letter 't' after a page number represents a table and 'f' represents a figure.